TEXTURE ANALYSIS IN MACHINE VISION

SERIES IN MACHINE PERCEPTION AND ARTIFICIAL INTELLIGENCE*

Editors: **H. Bunke** (Univ. Bern, Switzerland)
P. S. P. Wang (Northeastern Univ., USA)

*For the complete list of titles in this series, please write to the Publisher.

Series in Machine Perception and Artificial Intelligence – Vol. 40

TEXTURE ANALYSIS IN MACHINE VISION

Editor

M K Pietikäinen

University of Oulu, Finland

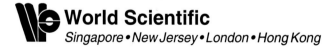

World Scientific

Singapore • New Jersey • London • Hong Kong

Published by

World Scientific Publishing Co. Pte. Ltd.

P O Box 128, Farrer Road, Singapore 912805

USA office: Suite 1B, 1060 Main Street, River Edge, NJ 07661

UK office: 57 Shelton Street, Covent Garden, London WC2H 9HE

British Library Cataloguing-in-Publication Data
A catalogue record for this book is available from the British Library.

TEXTURE ANALYSIS IN MACHINE VISION
Series in Machine Perception and Artificial Intelligence — Vol. 40

For photocopying of material in this volume, please pay a copying fee through the Copyright Clearance Center, Inc., 222 Rosewood Drive, Danvers, MA 01923, USA. In this case permission to photocopy is not required from the publisher.

ISBN 981-02-4373-1

Printed in Singapore by Uto-Print

CONTENTS

PREFACE

MATTI PIETIKÄINEN

Machine Vision and Media Processing Unit, Infotech Oulu
P.O. Box 4500, FIN-90014 University of Oulu, Finland
E-mail: mkp@ee.oulu.fi

Texture analysis is an important generic research area of machine vision. The potential areas of application include biomedical image analysis, industrial inspection, analysis of satellite or aerial imagery, content-based retrieval from image databases, document analysis, biometric person authentication, scene analysis for robot navigation, texture synthesis for computer graphics and animation, and image coding. Texture analysis has been a topic of intensive research for over three decades, but the progress has been very slow. The analysis of real world textures has turned out to be a very difficult problem, and there are only a limited number of examples of successful exploitation of texture.

A Workshop on Texture Analysis in Machine Vision was arranged at the University of Oulu, Finland, on June 14-15, 1999. The aim was to provide a forum for presenting recent research results and for discussing how to make progress in order to increase the usefulness of texture in practical applications. The program of the workshop included keynote presentations by professors Rama Chellappa (Univesity of Maryland, USA) and Anil K. Jain (Michigan State University, USA), contributed papers describing recent progress in this field, and a panel on future research directions.

This book contains extended and revised versions of the papers presented in the workshop. The first part of the book deals with texture analysis methodology, while the second part covers various applications.

In Chapter 1, Pietikäinen and Ojala present an overview of their nonparametric approach to texture analysis based on local binary patterns and signed gray-level differences. Rehrauer and Datcu then propose a scale selection algorithm based on a multi-scale random field model with a dynamic pyramidial structure. The paper from Mościńska and Tyma in Chapter 3 presents a two stage method for texture segmentation using estimated GMRF parameters for rough segmentation and neural networks for postprocessing.

In Chapter 4, Battiato and Gallo describe a nonparametric multiresolution approach for the analysis/synthesis of textures. A texture classification system using statistical and soft-computing methods is then proposed by Stolpmann and Dooley. Chapter 6, by Chetverikov and Földvári, considers the problem of affine-invariant texture classification using regularity features, and Soriano *et al.* deal with

vii

classification of tilted rough textures using local binary pattern operators. Finlayson and Tian discuss the results of a psychological study on color texture similarity. In Chapter 9, Botchko *et al.* propose an approach for virtual coloring of multispectral textures.

The second part of the book concerning applications begins with image retrieval and document analysis. In Chapter 10, Aksoy and Haralick consider both macro and micro aspects of texture in their approach to image similarity and retrieval. Leow and Lai propose a scale and orientation-invariant method for image retrieval based on Gabor filtering, and Okun and Pietikäinen present a survey on texture-based methods for document image analysis.

Applications in biomedical image analysis are considered in three papers. Chapter 13 by Yuen *et al.* deals with tongue texture analysis of traditional Chinese medicine using wavelet opponent color features. Materka *et al.* are concerned with analyzing X-ray images for the detection of bone mass and structure. In Chapter 15, Materka *et al.* consider texture analysis of test object (phantom) images for the standardization of *in vivo* magnetic resonance imaging.

Industrial inspection applications are represented by four papers. In Chapter 16, Silvén overviews the problems of applying texture analysis to industrial inspection. Schael and Burkhardt propose two methods for the automatic detection of errors on non-stochastic textures using invariant gray scale features and polynomial classifiers. In Chapter 18 Iivarinen presents a simple approach to surface defect segmentation based on local binary pattern texture measures and self-organizing map classification. Telfer describes a method for angular texture discrimination of woodgrain imagery using a directionally selective local feature statistics operator.

Finally, Chapter 20 by Ollila *et al.* combines the analysis and synthesis of textures with applications in the animation industry.

In summary, this book gives a unique view of different approaches and applications of texture analysis. It should be of great interest both to researchers of machine vision and to practitioners in various application areas.

I would like to thank all those whose contributions made this book possible, including the authors of the papers, the program and organizing committee members, and the reviewers of the workshop held in Oulu.

METHODOLOGY

NONPARAMETRIC TEXTURE ANALYSIS WITH COMPLEMENTARY SPATIAL OPERATORS

MATTI PIETIKÄINEN AND TIMO OJALA

Machine Vision and Media Processing Unit, Infotech Oulu
P.O. Box 4500, FIN-90014 University of Oulu, Finland
E-mail: {mkp,skidi}@ee.oulu.fi

Recently, we have developed a nonparametric approach to texture analysis, in which the distributions of simple texture measures based on local binary patterns and signed gray level differences are used to provide complementary information about the structural and stochastic properties of image texture. Very good performance has been obtained in various texture classification and segmentation problems. This paper overviews our approach and discusses reasons for its efficiency.

1 Introduction

Texture analysis is important in many applications of computer image analysis for classification, detection, or segmentation of images based on local spatial variations of intensity or color. Many different approaches to texture analysis have been proposed. Among the most widely used texture measures are those derived from gray level cooccurrence matrices or difference histograms, "texture energy" measures obtained by local linear transforms, features based on multi-channel Gabor filtering, wavelets, and Markov random field models [4,6,34,3].

Recently, we have developed a nonparametric approach to texture analysis, in which the distributions of simple texture measures based on local binary patterns and signed gray level differences are used to provide complementary information about the structural and stochastic properties of image texture. Very good performance has been obtained in various texture classification and segmentation problems, see e.g. [7,14-23,25-27,32]. This paper overviews our approach and discusses reasons for its efficiency.

2 Texture Description with Simple Spatial Operators

Consider the 3x3 neighborhood illustrated in Fig. 1, where g_i, i=0,...,8, denote the gray values of the respective pixels. We start the derivation of our texture operator by defining texture T as the joint distribution of the gray levels of the nine pixels:

$$T = p(g_0, g_1, g_2, g_3, g_4, g_5, g_6, g_7, g_8) \qquad (1)$$

3

g_4	g_2	g_3
g_5	g_0	g_1
g_6	g_7	g_8

Figure 1. A 3x3 neighborhood; g_i denotes the gray value of pixel i.

Without losing information, we can subtract the gray value of the center pixel from the gray values of the surrounding pixels:

$$T = p(g_0, g_1 - g_0, ..., g_8 - g_0) \qquad (2)$$

Assuming that the differences g_i-g_0 are independent of g_0, we can factorize Eq. (2):

$$T \sim p(g_0)p(g_1 - g_0, ..., g_8 - g_0) \qquad (3)$$

In practice an exact independence is not warranted, hence the factorized distribution is only an approximation of the joint distribution. However, we are willing to accept the possible small loss in information, as it allows us to achieve invariance with respect to shifts in gray scale. Namely, the distribution $p(g_0)$ in Eq. (3) describes the overall luminance of the image, which is unrelated to local image texture, and consequently does not provide useful information for texture analysis. Hence, much of the information in the original joint gray level distribution about the textural characteristics is conveyed by the joint difference distribution:

$$T \sim p(g_1 - g_0, ..., g_8 - g_0) \qquad (4)$$

2.1 Signed Gray-level Differences

Recently, Ojala et al. [23] showed that an approach based on multidimensional distributions of signed gray level differences of neighboring pixel values is very powerful for texture classification. The advantages of gray-level differences over the traditional co-occurrence method are: (1) the differences fall mainly within a narrower range than the gray levels due to the high correlation between gray levels of adjacent pixels, consequently providing a more compact description of texture;

(2) the signed differences are not affected by changes in mean luminance. In comparison to the commonly used absolute differences, the signed differences contain more information about image texture and consequently are more powerful.

In our experiments, the classification performance of two-, four-, and eight-dimensional difference distributions has been evaluated. By computing co-occurring differences within 3x3-pixel subimages (Fig. 1), we estimate the following distributions,

$$p_2(g_1 - g_0, g_2 - g_0) \tag{5}$$

$$p_4(g_1 - g_0, g_2 - g_0, g_3 - g_0, g_4 - g_0) \tag{6}$$

$$p_8(g_1 - g_0, g_2 - g_0, ..., g_8 - g_0) \tag{7}$$

The volume of the difference space for an image with G gray levels equals $(2G - 1)^k$, where $k=2,4,8$, corresponding to the distribution we are estimating. If we would straightforwardly describe the difference space with a k-dimensional histogram, we would obtain, even with modest values of G, very large histograms that are computationally expensive and suspect to statistical unreliability. Instead of reducing G, for example, with simple requantization of each co-ordinate, we partition the k-dimensional difference space using vector quantization [20]. For this purpose, we employ a codebook of N k-dimensional codewords, which have indices $n = 0,1,...,N-1$. The codebook is trained with the optimized LVQ1 training algorithm [11], by selecting random vectors from each of the samples in the training set. Our method of vector quantization is computationally much simpler than that used by Valkealahti and Oja [35].

We describe the difference information of a texture sample with a difference histogram. The mapping from the difference space to a difference histogram is straightforward. Given a particular k-dimensional difference vector, the index of the nearest codeword corresponds to the bin index in the difference histogram. In other words, a codebook of N codewords produces a histogram of N bins. The difference histogram of a texture sample is obtained by searching the nearest codeword to each vector present in the sample, and incrementing the bin denoted by the index of this nearest codeword.

2.2 Local Binary Patterns

Signed differences are not affected by changes in mean luminance, hence they are invariant against gray scale shifts. We achieve invariance with respect to the scaling of the gray scale by considering just the signs of the differences instead of their exact values:

$$T \sim p(s(g_1 - g_0),...,s(g_8 - g_0)) \tag{8}$$

where

$$s(x) = \begin{cases} 1, x \geq 0 \\ 0, x \prec 0 \end{cases} \tag{9}$$

If we formulate Eq. (8) slightly differently, we obtain the LBP (Local Binary Pattern) operator introduced by Ojala et al. [19]:

$$LBP = \sum_{i=1}^{8} s(g_i - g_0)2^{i-1} \tag{10}$$

The computation of LBP is illustrated in Fig. 2. The original 3x3 neighborhood is thresholded by the value of the center pixel. The values of the pixels in the thresholded neighborhood are multiplied by the binomial weights given to the corresponding pixels. Finally, the values of the eight pixels are summed to obtain the LBP number for this neighborhood.

example			thresholded			weights		
6	5	2	1	0	0	1	2	4
7	6	1	1		0	128		8
9	8	7	1	1	1	64	32	16

Pattern = **11110001**
LBP = 1 + 16 +32 + 64 + 128 =   **241**
C = (6+7+8+9+7)/5 - (5+2+1)/3 =   **4.7**

Figure 2. Computation of Local Binary Pattern (LBP) and contrast measure C.

LBP can be regarded as a simplification of p_8. It is obvious that LBP contains less textural information than p_8. The motivation for using LBP instead of p_8 is two-fold: LBP's gray scale invariance and computational simplicity. Effectively, whereas signed differences measure both the spatial organization (pattern) and the contrast (amount) of local image texture, with LBP we intentionally focus only on spatial structure and discard contrast, as it depends on the gray scale.

LBP is by definition invariant against any monotonic transformation of the gray scale, i.e. as long as the order of pixel values stays the same, the output of the LBP operator remains constant. This makes LBP very attractive in situations where the gray scale is subject to changes due to, for example, varying illumination conditions which often have to be coped with in many applications, e.g. in visual inspection. Computational simplicity is another obvious advantage, as there is no need for the quantization of the feature space or other time consuming computations, but the easily calculated 8-bit LBP numbers are simply accumulated into a histogram of 256 bins. This results in a very straightforward and efficient implementation, which may come in handy in time critical applications.

As we noted earlier, LBP does not address the contrast of texture which is important in the discrimination of some textures. For this purpose, we can combine LBP with a simple contrast measure C as shown in Fig. 2 and consider joint occurrences of LBP and C.

He and Wang [8] introduced the Texture Unit operator, which is similar to LBP, but it uses three levels (i.e. two thresholds) instead of two levels used in LBP. This leads to a more inefficient representation and implementation than with LBP (6561 bin values instead of 256), and according to our tests the three-level operator does not perform any better than LBP. The Texture Unit operator usually also needs a user defined delta value for setting the threshold values, which makes it dependent on the gray scale variance.

LBP encodes various simple feature detectors (edge, curve/line, corner, curve/line end, spot/flatness) at different orientations in a single operator. The LBP histogram contains the density of each feature over a given region. An important point is that for each pixel the output of the best-matching feature detector is only utilized. A conventional texture analysis method based on spatial filtering (e.g., Laws' masks, Gabor filters) creates a feature vector for each pixel containing information from both relevant and irrelevant local pattern matches, making this kind of approach less efficient.

Some may find the performance of LBP surprisingly good, given the small support of 3x3 pixels. One may argue that this operator size is by no means adequate, in comparison to the much larger Gabor filter masks that are often used., for example. Actually, the 'built-in' support of the operator is inherently larger than 3x3 pixels, as only a specific limited set of binary patterns can occur next to a particular binary pattern. Further, the histogram of local operator responses incorporates larger scale texture properties. However, if a larger scale analysis is required, it can be accomplished simply by increasing the predicate (i.e. neighborhood size) of the operator. This means that we choose the eight neighbors of the center pixel from the corresponding positions in different neighborhoods (3x3, 5x5, 7x7, etc.) [15].

3   Experiments with Texture Classification

The 32 Brodatz textures used in the experiments are shown in Fig. 3 [2,35]. The images are 256x256 pixels in size and they have 256 gray levels. Each image was divided into 16 disjoint 64x64 samples, which were independently histogram-equalized to remove luminance differences between textures. To make the classification problem more challenging and generic, three additional samples were generated from each sample: a sample rotated by 90 degrees, a 64x64 scaled sample obtained from the 45x45 pixels in the middle of the 'original' sample, and a sample that was both rotated and scaled. Consequently, the classification problem involved a total of 2048 samples, 64 samples in each of the 32 texture categories [35].

The texture classifier was trained by randomly choosing, in each texture class, eight 'original' samples, together with the corresponding 24 transformed samples, as models. The other half of the data, eight 'original' samples and the corresponding 24 transformed samples in each texture class, was used for testing the classifier. In the classification phase a test sample S was assigned to the class of the model M that maximized the log-likelihood measure:

$$L(S, M) = \sum_{n=1}^{N} S_n \ln M_n \qquad (11)$$

where S_n and M_n correspond to the sample and model probabilities of bin n, respectively.

We estimated distributions p_2, p_4 and p_8, by partitioning the difference space with a codebook of 384 codewords. The codebook was trained with the standard optimized LVQ1 training algorithm, by selecting 100 random vectors from each of the 1024 samples in the training set.

In experiments, we obtained classification accuracies of 93.3% for p_2, 95.7% for p_4 and 96.8% for p_8, respectively [23]. These results are excellent considering the difficulty of the problem. The simple LBP operator achieved an accuracy of 91.2%, i.e. about 5 % less than the much more complex p_8 operator.

For comparison, experiments were carried out with features based on standard GMRF models and Gabor filtering using different mask sizes, with the same implementation as in the MeasTex site [31]. Two different classifiers, the k nearest neighbor classifier and the multivariate Gaussian discriminant, were used for classification. The best result for the GRMF approach was 77.0%, obtained with a standard 6th order symmetric mask and the multivariate Gaussian discriminant classifier. The best combination of GMRF features obtained from features computed using all models from the 1st order to the 7th order achieved 89.3%. The best standard Gabor features, extracted with a filter bank of three different wavelengths and four different orientations in a 11x11 neighborhood and using the Gaussian discriminant classifier, achieved an accuracy of 90.0%. The best combination of Gabor features obtained from features computed using all mask sizes between 3x3 and 19x19 pixels achieved an accuracy of 91.8%. We were able to improve the accuracy of the Gabor approach from these figures by using both the means and standard deviations of the magnitudes of the filtered images together as texture features, instead of using only the means, as is normally the case. The 'optimized' filter design strategy of Manjunath and Ma [13] also improved the results.

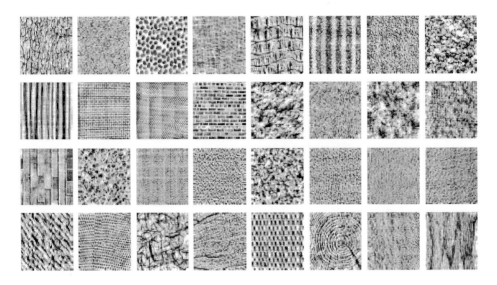

Figure 3. Brodatz textures used in classification experiments.

As we can see, these computationally complex methods used in comparisons performed poorer than our simple methods, even though a larger neighborhood was used to compute the features, instead of the 3x3 neighborhood used in our approach. The rather poor results obtained with the GMRF method are partly caused by the histogram equalization that was used to remove the effects of unequal global brightness and contrast.

4   Experiments with Unsupervised Texture Segmentation

Recently, an unsupervised texture segmentation algorithm using the LBP/C texture measure and nonparametric statistical test was developed by Ojala and Pietikäinen [18]. The method has performed very well in experiments. It is not sensitive to the selection of parameter values, does not require any prior knowledge about the number of textures or regions in the image as most existing approaches do, and seems to provide significantly better results than existing approaches. The method can be easily generalized, e.g., to utilize other texture features, multiscale information, color features, and combinations of multiple features.

The segmentation method consists of three phases: hierarchical splitting, agglomerative merging and pixelwise classification. First, hierarchical splitting is used to divide the image into regions of roughly uniform texture. Then, an agglomerative merging procedure merges similar adjacent regions until a stopping criterion is met. At this point, we have obtained rough estimates of the different textured regions present in the image, and we complete the analysis by a pixelwise classification to improve the localization. Fig. 4 illustrates the steps of the segmentation algorithm on a 512 x 512 mosaic containing five different Brodatz textures.

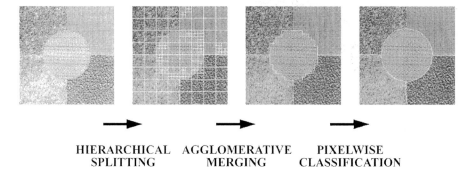

HIERARCHICAL   AGGLOMERATIVE   PIXELWISE
   SPLITTING   MERGING   CLASSIFICATION

Figure 4. Main sequence of the segmentation algorithm.

We have applied our segmentation method to a variety of texture mosaics with excellent results [18,9]. The database in [9] was created from a set of 86 textures from the Brodatz album, by constructing 100 random mixtures (512x512 pixels each) of five textures. Puzicha et al. [29] detected the overall structure of the mosaic correctly (i.e. the percentage of mislabeled pixels was below 20%) in 95 cases with their ACM (asymmetric clustering model) based multiscale segmentation algorithm when the number of textures was manually provided. The median segmentation error (i.e. the proportion of mislabeled pixels) of all 100 cases was 2.8%, when a topological prior eliminating unlikely label configurations in small neighborhoods was incorporated. Our unsupervised algorithm, which tries to detect the number of textures by itself, found the correct structure in 81 cases, when the minimum region size in hierarchical splitting was set to 32x32 pixels. The median segmentation error of all 100 cases was 2.3%. The 19 failures occurred with mixtures that contained large-scale texture(s), whose dominating texture pattern was too large to be captured by the 3x3 neighborhood of the LBP/C operator used in our algorithm. This calls for a multiscale approach, where outputs of LBP/C operators computed at different scales are utilized.

The segmentation of a natural scene taken from [24] is shown in Fig. 5 [18]. The textures of natural scenes are generally more non-uniform than the homogeneous textures of the test mosaics. Also, in natural scenes adjacent textured regions are not necessarily separated by well-defined boundaries, but the spatial pattern smoothly changes from one texture to another. Further, we have to observe the infinite scale of texture differences present in natural scenes; choosing the right scale is a very subjective matter. For these reasons there is often no 'correct' segmentation for a natural scene, as is the case with texture mosaics.

The invariance of the LBP/C transform to average luminance shows in the bottom part of the image, where the sea is interpreted as a single region despite the shadows. The result obtained is very satisfactory, considering that important color or gray scale information is not utilized in the segmentation.

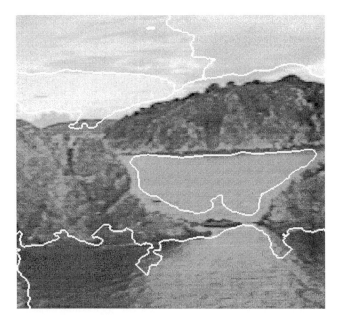

Figure 5. Segmentation of a natural scene.

5 Recent developments

In their recent paper, Randen and Husøy reviewed the filtering approaches to texture feature extraction and performed an extensive comparative study using an image set of twelve different types of mosaics of varying complexity [30]. For comparison, the co-occurrence and multiresolution autoregressive (AR) features were also included in the study. In their experiments, various filtering approaches yielded different results for different images. No single approach performed best or very close to the best for all images. The computational complexity of the methods was also considered to be too high. Randen and Husøy concluded that a very useful direction for future research is the development of powerful texture measures that can be extracted and classified with low computational complexity.

We benchmarked the LBP and signed gray level difference approaches in supervised texture segmentation using the same image set as Randen and Husøy and following their experimental setup as closely as possible [23]. The results were excellent. The best signed difference or LBP operator outperformed the best result from Randen and Husøy in 11 of the 12 cases, and in most cases by a clear margin. The LBP approach, despite its simplicity, provided the lowest error rate of all operators in seven of the 12 cases, and the signed gray level difference in four cases, respectively. The impressive result of LBP can largely be attributed to its gray scale invariance. It is understandably a very useful property when the gray scale properties of the unknown test sample differ from the training data, which appeared to be the case in most of the images used in this study.

Recently, we also proposed a simple multiscale extension for LBP by using simultaneously multiple LBP operators computed with different neighborhood sizes [15]. With this approach, the performance of LBP was further improved, indicating that in most cases it is advantageous to use more than just one predicate for the LBP operator. Additionally, we have been developing a multichannel version for color texture analysis, where the computation of LBP is based on an opponent color type representation.

Considering the texture primitive interpretation of LBP as discussed in Section 2.2, it is obvious that all 256 encoded patterns are not equally important. Some patterns should remain more stable under geometric transformations and thus perform better in classification. We have demonstrated that a small subset of local patterns encoded in LBP can perfom better than the whole histogram in problems involving geometric transformation between training and testing images [14].

A related obervation is that a small subset of 'uniform' local binary patterns with no or a minimal number of spatial $0 \rightarrow 1$ (or $1 \rightarrow 0$) transitions along the circularly symmetric neighborhood of the 8 surrounding pixels appears to sustain rotation very well. Very impressive results were obtained in our recent study on rotation and gray scale invariant texture classification, in which occurrence statistics of these rotation-invariant 'uniform' patterns were used for discrimination [21]. The use of 'uniform' patterns means that we ignore 'nonuniform' patterns which, by having a larger number of spatial transitions, are more vulnerable to unwanted changes upon rotation. This approximation is supported by the fact that the 'uniform' patterns seem to contribute the majority of the local patterns present in Brodatz, like deterministic microtextures, sometimes up to 95%. Further improvement was achieved by quantizing the angular space at a finer resolution (22.5°) than in the original LBP (45°). This kind of operator used in conjunction with a local variance measure outperfomed the existing rotation-invariant texture measures for the same test images that were used in recent papers [5,27,28].

This notion of using a subset of all available patterns can be extended further into determining a problem or application specific set of patterns, which provides the best performance. However, there is a danger that the chosen subset becomes too specialized to the training data, and does not generalize properly to unknown testing data.

6   Discussion

The role of local features (primitives, textural elements, textons) and their differences in preattentive texture discrimination has been established in psychophysical studies [1,10]. Our approach fits in well with these findings: simple feature detectors are used to measure perceptually significant textural properties and the segmentation is performed by comparing textural similarities of neighboring regions on the basis of densities of different features.

In our approach, the distributions of texture measures based on local binary patterns and signed gray level differences are used to provide complementary information about the structural and stochastic properties of image texture, making it very efficient for various types of micro- and macrotextures.

The texture primitives detected by LBP could be linked to more complex textural elements using principles of proximity and good continuation, but our excellent results suggest that this is usually not so important. Coarseness, edge orientation and contrast are perceptually very important textural properties [33,12]. The LBP histograms contain information about edge orientation and coarseness (e.g. edges per unit area). LBP does not address the contrast of texture. For this purpose, we can combine LBP with a simple contrast measure C. This measure is invariant with respect to average luminance, which is very important considering, for example, the needs of texture segmentation (see Fig. 5).

LBP is invariant against any monotonic gray scale transformation, which is a necessary property in many applications involving uneven illumination or great within-class variability; see, for example, our results in metal strip inspection [25] and in the classification of tilted 3D textures [32]. The basic LBP method is sensitive to texture orientation, but this property appears to be very useful in texture segmentation, e.g. for finding accurate boundaries between neighboring regions. A rotation invariant version of LBP was proposed in [16,27], but recently we have significantly improved it by concentrating only on a subset of rotation invariant patterns encoded in LBP and by quantizing the angular space at a finer resolution [21].

The signed gray level difference method is closely related to the widely used co-occurence method. It is invariant with respect to average luminance, while the co-occurrence approach is not. The method is highly efficient in applications involving stochastic textures, but it also discriminates more structured textures very well. The difference histograms provide information about the coarseness and contrast of texture. For a coarse texture, the difference histogram will peak near zero, but for a finer-grained texture it will spread out more uniformly. The eight-dimensional signed gray level difference operator can be regarded as a generalization of the LBP operator, capturing information about both structural and stochastic aspects of texture.

The importance of the spatial pattern and contrast information in texture discrimination is also supported by our other findings. A joint pair of a rotation-invariant version of LBP and a local variance measure provided the best performance in our experiments with rotation-invariant texture classification [27,21]. In addition, the original LBP measure and a measure based on absolute gray level differences were the best features for two different test image sets in our experiments with multichannel texture description, providing together nearly as good performance as an 'optimal' combination of all 12 measures used in the study [17].

The choice of highly discriminating texture features is very important for success in texture segmentation. The features should easily discriminate various types of textures, and the window size used for computing textural features should be small enough to be useful for small image regions and to provide small error rates at region boundaries. The LBP, LBP/C and signed gray level difference features perform well also for small image regions (e.g., 16 x 16 pixels), unlike many other approaches.

Local texture similarity can be measured very efficiently and reliably with a nonparametric statistical test as in our segmentation procedure. One major advantage is that these methods do not require the specification of a suitable vector-space metric. Similarity is instead defined directly via the respective feature distributions [9].

7   Conclusion

A nonparametric approach to texture analysis using simple spatial operators has been developed. The distributions of texture measures based on local binary patterns and signed gray level differences are used to provide complementary information about the strurctural and stochastic properties of image texture. Local texture similarity is measured very efficiently and reliably with nonparametric statistical tests. Our methodology resembles some well-known psychophysical models on human texture perception. The approach has provided excellent results in various texture classification and segmentation problems, and leads to computationally simple implementations. Our results should therefore be of great interest from both the theoretical and practical viewpoints when trying to find solutions that could increase the usefulness of texture in real-world applications.

8   Acknowledgements

The financial support provided by the Academy of Finland and the National Technology Agency (Teles) is gratefully acknowledged.

9   Note

Most of the image data used in our papers can be downloaded from *http://www.ee.oulu.fi/research/imag/texture.*

10   References

1. J. Beck, S. Prazdny and A. Rosenfeld, "A theory of textural segmentation," in *Human and Machine Vision*, eds. J. Beck, B. Hope and A. Rosenfeld, Academic, New York, 1983.
2. P. Brodatz, *Textures: A Photographic Album for Artists and Designers*, Dover Publications, New York, 1966.
3. R. Chellappa, R.L Kashyap and B.S. Manjunath, "Model-based texture segmentation and classification," in *Handbook of Pattern Recognition and Computer Vision, Second Edition*, eds. C.H. Chen, L.F. Pau, P.S.P. Wang, World Scientific, Singapore, 1999, pp. 249-282.
4. L. Van Gool, P. Dewaele and A. Oosterlinck, "Texture analysis anno 1983," *Comput. Vision Graph. Image Process.* 29 (1985) 336-357.

5. G.M. Haley and B.S. Manjunath, "Rotation-invariant texture classification using a complete space-frequency model," *IEEE Trans. Image Process.* 8 (1999) 255-269.
6. R.M. Haralick and L.G. Shapiro, *Computer and Robot Vision, Vol. 1*, Addison-Wesley, 1992.
7. D. Harwood, T. Ojala, M. Pietikäinen, S. Kelman and L. Davis, "Texture classification by center-symmetric autocorrelation, using Kullback discrimination of distributions," *Pattern Recogn. Lett.* 16 (1995) 1-10.
8. D.C. He and L. Wang, "Texture unit, texture spectrum and texture analysis," *IEEE Trans. Geosci. Remote Sensing* 28 (1990) 509-512.
9. T. Hofmann, J. Puzicha and J.M. Buhmann, "Unsupervised texture segmentation in a deterministic annealing framework," *IEEE Trans. Pattern Anal. Mach. Intell.* 20 (1998) 803-818.
10. B. Julesz and J.R. Bergen, "Textons, the fundamental elements in preattentive vision and perception of textures," *The Bell Syst. Techn. J.* 62 (1983) 1619-1645.
11. T. Kohonen, J. Kangas, J. Laaksonen and K. Torkkola, "LVQ_PAK: A program package for the correct application of learning vector quantization algorithms," *Proc. Int. Joint Conf. on Neural Networks*, Baltimore, 1992, pp. 1725-1730.
12. M. Levine, *Vision in Man and Machine*, McGraw-Hill, 1985.
13. B.S. Manjunath and W.Y. Ma, "Texture features for browsing and retrieval of image data, " *IEEE Trans. Pattern Anal. Mach. Intell.* 18 (1996) 837-842.
14. T. Mäenpää, T. Ojala, M. Pietikäinen and M. Soriano, "Robust texture classification by subsets of Local Binary Patterns," *Proc. 15th Int. Conf. on Pattern Recognition*, Barcelona, Spain 2000, in press.
15. T. Mäenpää, M. Pietikäinen and T. Ojala, "Texture classification by multi-predicate Local Binary Pattern operators," *Proc. 15th Int. Conf. on Pattern Recognition*, 2000, in press.
16. T. Ojala, Nonparametric Texture Analysis Using Simple Spatial Operators, with Applications in Visual Inspection, *Acta Univ. Ouluensis*, C 105, 1997.
17. T. Ojala and M. Pietikäinen, "Nonparametric multichannel texture description with simple spatial operators," *Proc. 14th Int. Conf. on Pattern Recognition*, Brisbane, Australia, 1998, pp. 1952-1056.
18. T. Ojala and M. Pietikäinen, "Unsupervised texture segmentation using feature distributions," *Pattern Recogn.* 32 (1999) 477-486.
19. T. Ojala, M. Pietikäinen and D. Harwood, "A comparative study of texture measures with classification based on feature distributions," *Pattern Recogn.* 29 (1996) 51-59.
20. T. Ojala, M. Pietikäinen and J. Kyllönen, "Gray level cooccurrence histograms via learning vector quantization," *Proc. 11th Scand. Conf. on Image Analysis*, Kangerlussuaq, Greenland, 1999, pp. 103-108.

21. T. Ojala and M. Pietikäinen and T. Mäenpää, "Gray scale and rotation invariant texture classification with Local Binary Patterns," *Proc. Sixth European Conf. on Computer Vision*, Dublin, Ireland, 2000, in press.

22. T. Ojala, M. Pietikäinen and J. Nisula, "Determining composition of grain mixtures by texture classification based on feature distributions," *Int. J. Pattern Recogn. Artif. Intell.* 10 (1996) 73-82.

23. T. Ojala, K. Valkealahti, E. Oja and M. Pietikäinen, "Texture discrimination with multidimensional distributions of signed gray level differences," *Pattern Recogn. (2000)*, in press.

24. D.K. Panjwani and G. Healey, "Markov random field models for unsupervised segmentation of textured color images," *IEEE Trans. Pattern Anal. Mach. Intell.* 17 (1995) 939-954.

25. M. Pietikäinen, T. Ojala, J. Nisula and J. Heikkinen, "Experiments with two industrial problems using texture classification based on feature distributions," *SPIE 2354 Intelligent Robots and Computer Vision XIII: 3D Vision, Product Inspection and Active Vision*, 1994, pp. 197-204.

26. M. Pietikäinen, T. Ojala and O. Silven, "Approaches to texture-based classification, segmentation and surface inspection," in *Handbook of Pattern Recognition and Computer Vision, Second Edition*, eds. C.H. Chen, L.F. Pau, P.S.P. Wang, World Scientific, Singapore, 1999, pp. 711-736.

27. M. Pietikäinen, T. Ojala and Z. Xu, "Rotation-invariant texture classification using feature distributions," *Pattern Recogn. 33* (2000), 43-52.

28. R. Porter and N. Canagarajah, "Robust rotation-invariant texture classification: wavelet, Gabor filter and GMRF based schemes," *IEE Proc. Vision Image Signal Process.* 144 (1997) 180-188.

29. J. Puzicha, T. Hofmann and J.M. Buhmann, "Histogram clustering for unsupervised segmentation and image retrieval," *Pattern Recogn. Lett.* 20 (1999) 899-909.

30. T. Randen and J.H. Husøy, "Filtering for texture classification: a comparative study, " *IEEE Trans. Pattern Anal. Mach. Intell.* 21 (1999), 291-310. *http:// www.ux.his.no/~tranden/*.

31. G. Smith and I. Burns, "Measuring texture classification algorithms," *Pattern Recogn. Lett.* 18 (1997) 1495-1501. http://www.cssip.elec.uq.edu.au/~guy/meastex/meastex.html.

32. M. Soriano, T. Ojala and M. Pietikäinen, "Robustness of Local Binary Pattern (LBP) operators to tilt-compensated textures", in *Texture Analysis in Machine Vision*, ed. M. Pietikäinen, World Scientific, Singapore, 2000.

33. H. Tamura, S. Mori and T. Yamawaki, "Textural features corresponding to visual perception," *IEEE Trans. Syst. Man Cybern.* 8 (1978) 460-473.

34. M. Tuceryan and A.K. Jain, "Texture analysis," in *Handbook of Pattern Recognition and Computer Vision, Second Edition*, eds. C.H. Chen, L.F. Pau, P.S.P. Wang, World Scientific, Singapore, 1999, pp. 207-248.

35. K. Valkealahti and E. Oja, "Reduced multidimensional cooccurrence histograms in texture classification," *IEEE Trans. Pattern Anal. Mach. Intell.* 20 (1998) 90-94.

SELECTING SCALES FOR TEXTURE MODELS

HUBERT REHRAUER

Communication Technology Lab, Image Science Group,
Swiss Federal Institute of Technology, ETH Zürich, Gloriastr. 35, CH-8092 Zürich
E-mail: rehrauer@vision.ee.ethz.ch

MIHAI DATCU

German Aerospace Center DLR, German Remote Sensing Data Center DFD,
D-82234 Wessling
E-mail: mihai.datcu@dlr.de

Texture models are widely in use for image content description. If textures occur at very different scales elaborated multi-scale approaches are required. This paper presents a scale selection method which estimates the most appropriate scales of the image data for texture analysis. The model is based on a multi-scale random field with a dynamic pyramidal structure. It can be used as a preprocessing step of a texture analysis indicating the scales and regions that are relevant for the analysis. The model helps to reduce the number of features to be used for image characterization while maintaining a good classification performance.

1 Introduction

Visual information in images is often present in the form of texture. Texture models extract the information contained in the spatial variations of the image data. In many images and especially in remote-sensing data, textures are present at very different scales. This means that, independent of the scale of the image, we will always perceive some texture. However the texture and its interpretation are dependent on the scale. In remote-sensing images a fine scale texture may originate, for example, from a vegetation pattern on agricultural fields. The fact that these fields are situated in a large valley surrounded by hills is not encoded in the fine-scale texture. To detect this we have to analyze the texture at a coarse scale. Information extraction based on textures should reflect this.

Popular approaches for texture classification are filtering methods and Markov random field (MRF) models (see the comparison paper of Randen [1] for an overview). These are based on kernels of a certain size. Additionally the estimation is done within windows of again a limited size. As a consequence these models are only efficient if the wavelength of the intensity variations lies within a certain spatial range which is constrained by the size of the model's kernel and the size of the estimation window.

Information extraction from images using such "single scale" texture models can be enhanced if the texture models are embedded in a multi-scale frame [2] [3]. A complete description of all textures present in the data requires either the running of a texture model with different kernel sizes on the same data, or the running of a texture model with a fixed kernel size on scaled versions of the data. Both approaches are computationally costly. Additionally they result in a high dimensional index that is difficult to interpret. Alternatively there exist intrinsic multi-scale texture models like the multi-resolution simultaneous auto regression model (MRSAR) by Mao and Jain [4] or the multi-scale random field model by Luettgen et al. [5]. In these models texture parameters are always related to a certain scale of the texture. These approaches are again computationally demanding and produce a rather high-dimensional feature vector.

The goal of scale selection is to use the advantages of multi-scale feature extractors but to avoid too complex a description of the data. Using the fact that the data often exhibit significant spatial variations only at certain scales, which we call the "characteristic" scales of the data, a scale selection is made and texture parameters are used only at those scales. This reduces the computational load drastically without loosing the descriptive power.

A different approach to scale selection has been proposed by Lindeberg [6]. His approach is based on the scale space theory in image processing [7] which gives the rules for the construction of multi-scale representations of images and spatial data in general. Within this theory various feature extraction methods at continuous scales are available. Recently, it was shown how they can be combined with a scale selection algorithm based on normalized spatial derivatives [6]. However this works only for special features like edges, ridges and blobs, and not for texture in general. These features are computed on multiple scales and then the scale that gives the best representation is selected.

Our approach is to provide a scheme for scale selection in texture analysis that serves as a *fast* preprocessing step to evaluate the characteristic scales of the image. The scale selection is based on a multi-scale random field model with a pyramidal structure. The layers of the pyramid correspond to the dyadic scales. We adapt the inter scale statistical dependencies of the random variables to the data and we make a maximum a-posteriori estimation of the field and the inter scale transition probability distributions. The characteristic scales are computed from the variance of the transition probability density function (PDF).

The scheme has been developed for the upcoming content-based retrieval system of the Swiss Remote Sensing Image Archive [8]. Queries for image content are based on multi-scale families of precomputed signal-oriented indices

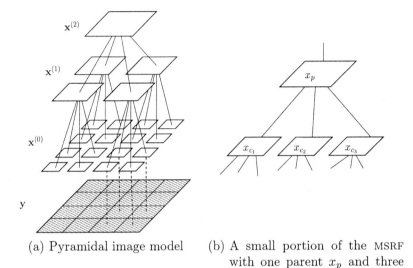

(a) Pyramidal image model

(b) A small portion of the MSRF with one parent x_p and three children $x_{c_1}, x_{c_2}, x_{c_3}$.

Figure 1. Multi-scale random field

that characterize the images. The scale selection indicates for an unknown cover-type class the optimum scale for the characterization.

In the next section we give the mathematical foundation of the model and present the algorithm for scale selection. Sec. 3 shows results on homogeneous texture images and gives an application example from our content-based retrieval system.

2   Scale selection model

A pyramidal multi-scale random field (MSRF) model[a] serves as image model for the scale selection. Fig. 1(a) sketches the image model. Each layer $\mathbf{x}^{(l)}, l = 0, \ldots, L - 1$ of the pyramid is a field of random variables (RVs) situated on a 2D lattice $S^{(l)}$.

$$\mathbf{x}^{(l)} = \{x_i \,|\, x_i \in S^{(l)}\}$$

All RVs of the pyramid are indexed by a scalar index. The layer or scale l of the pyramid corresponds to the dyadic scale 2^l relative to the scale of the

---

[a]The MSRF can also be described by the theory of Bayesian belief networks [9].

data. The connections of the RVs show the only conditional dependencies among them. At the bottom there is the image **y** that is "emitted" by the base layer of the pyramid $\mathbf{x}^{(0)}$ with one RV of the base layer associated to each image pixel.

The model as shown in Fig. 1 (a) is identical to the quadtree model proposed for image segmentation by Bouman and Shapiro [10]. We extend this model in that we allow the conditional dependencies to switch, thereby making the structure of the pyramid dynamic. We have presented this type of MSRF already in the frame of multi-scale image segmentation [11].

Given the image **y** we estimate the maximum a posteriori (MAP) configuration of the pyramid. The configuration of the pyramid comprises the *inter scale connections*, the *transition probability density functions* and the *maximum a posteriori states* of the RVs. We find the MAP configuration by a two-step iterative procedure. In a *fine-to-coarse* step, we estimate the state and transition PDFs, and in a *coarse-to-fine* step, we maximize the MAP probability by choosing the appropriate states and dependencies. The iteration stops when a local maximum of the MAP probability of the pyramid is reached. The "characteristic" scales result from an analysis of the transition PDFs of the MAP-configuration.

2.1 Properties of the MSRF pyramid

The basic properties of the pyramid are Markovianity across scale

$$P[\mathbf{x}^{(l)} | \mathbf{x}^{(l')}, l' \geq l] = P[\mathbf{x}^{(l)} | \mathbf{x}^{(l+1)}] \tag{1}$$

and independence of neighboring variables given the variables at the next coarser scale

$$P[x_i, x_j | \mathbf{x}^{(l+1)}] = P[x_i | \mathbf{x}^{(l+1)}] P[x_j | \mathbf{x}^{(l+1)}] \quad i, j \in S^{(l)}. \tag{2}$$

The total probability of the MSRF and the image is

$$P[\mathbf{y}, \{\mathbf{x}^{(l)}\}] = P[\mathbf{y} | \mathbf{x}^{(0)}] P[\mathbf{x}^{(0)} | \mathbf{x}^{(1)}] \cdots P[\mathbf{x}^{(L-2)} | \mathbf{x}^{(L-1)}] P[\mathbf{x}^{(L-1)}]. \tag{3}$$

Due to the property (2) the transition and emission probabilities do factorize

$$P[\mathbf{x}^{(l)} | \mathbf{x}^{(l+1)}] = \prod_{i \in S^{(l)}} P[x_i | x_{\mathcal{P}(i)}]$$

$$P[\mathbf{y} | \mathbf{x}^{(0)}] = \prod_{i \in S^{(0)}} P[y_i | x_i]$$

with the parent operator $\mathcal{P}(\cdot) : \mathcal{P}(i) \in S^{(l+1)} \forall i \in S^{(l)}$ that returns the parent index. We assume Gaussian functions as PDFs for both the transition and the emission process.

Given the image $\mathbf{y}$ we estimate the posterior PDFs at the base layer. For each pixel i of the image we assume a Gaussian distribution of the gray values with the state of the base RV x_i as mean and the variance σ_i^2. We denote this by

$$P[y_i \,|\, x_i] = \mathcal{N}\left(y_i - x_i, \, \sigma_i^2\right), \quad i \in S^{(0)} \tag{4}$$

where the variance is estimated from the neighborhood ∂i of the pixel i

$$\sigma_i^2 = \frac{1}{|\partial i|} \sum_{j \in \partial i} (y_j - y_i)^2.$$

With a flat prior probability $P[x_i] = \text{const}$, the posterior PDF of the random variable x_i is

$$P[x_i \,|\, y_i] = \mathcal{N}\left(x_i - y_i, \, \sigma_i^2\right), \quad i \in S^{(0)}. \tag{5}$$

Starting from these posterior PDFs of the base layer we search the MAP configuration of the pyramid.

2.2   Fine-to-coarse step

We illustrate the algorithm on a node shown in Fig. 1(b). In this case the number of children N of the RV x_p equals to three, but the following equations are valid for an arbitrary number of children. The transition PDF from a parent to a child is modeled as a Gaussian distribution with zero mean and variance θ_p^2, and is identical for all children x_{c_n} of the parent x_p, so that the PDF of a child is given by

$$P[x_{c_n} \,|\, x_p] = \mathcal{N}\left(x_{c_n} - x_p, \, \theta_p^2\right), \quad n = 1, 2, 3. \tag{6}$$

Using the independence (2) and the Markovian property (1) we compute the posterior probabilities of the variables at the higher layers. We assume again a flat prior probability for the parent variable x_p and use Bayes' rule to write the posterior probability of the parent given the children $x_{c_1}, x_{c_2}, x_{c_3}$

$$P[x_p \,|\, \{x_{c_n}\}] \propto \prod_{n=1}^{N} \mathcal{N}\left(x_p - x_{c_n}, \, \theta_p^2\right) \tag{7}$$

which is a Gaussian. The posterior probability of the parent variable given the image is given by a product over all childen and the sum over all values of the children

$$P[x_p | \mathbf{y}] = \prod_{n=1}^{N} \sum_{x_{c_n}} P[x_p | x_{c_n}, \mathbf{y}] \, P[x_{c_n} | \mathbf{y}], \tag{8}$$

so that the posterior of the parent can be computed recursively from posteriors of the children. Assuming $P[x_{c_n} | \mathbf{y}] = \mathcal{N}\left(x_{c_n} - \mu_{c_n}, \sigma_{c_n}^2\right)$ and using the properties of Gaussian functions given in the Appendix, we derive that the posterior of the parent is a Gaussian

$$P[x_p | \mathbf{y}] = \mathcal{N}\left(x_p - \mu_p, \sigma_p^2\right), \tag{9}$$

with

$$\mu_p = \frac{1}{N} \sum_n \mu_{c_n} \tag{10}$$

$$\sigma_p^2 = \frac{N \theta_p^2 + \sum_n \sigma_{c_n}^2}{N^2} \tag{11}$$

From the mean values we estimate the transition parameters:

$$\theta_p^2 = \frac{1}{N} \sum_n (\mu_p - \mu_{c_n})^2 \tag{12}$$

The equations (10) (11) and (12) give the fine-to-coarse recursion formulas for the means and variances that determine the posterior PDFs of all variables in the pyramid.

The equations state that the mean of the parent PDF is the average of the means of its children. While the variance of the parent PDF has a contribution from the children's variances *and* the transition variance.

2.3   Coarse-to-fine step

In a second step that goes from coarse-to-fine we select the maximum a posteriori states $\hat{x}_i$ hierarchically. At the coarsest scale we have

$$\hat{x}_i = \mu_i, \quad i \in S^{(L-1)}$$

For all lower scales $l = L - 2, \ldots, 0$, we maximize the probability of the pyramid by selecting the optimal state and the *optimal parent*,

$$\hat{x}_i = \arg \max_{x_i, \, p \in \partial \mathcal{P}(i)} \mathcal{N}\left(x_i - \mu_i, \sigma_i^2\right) \mathcal{N}\left(x_i - \hat{x}_p, \theta_p^2\right) \qquad i \in S^{(l)} \tag{13}$$

Candidates for the parent are the four nearest neighbors at the next coarse scale. Although we start with an initial quadtree, the pyramid adapts after some iterations its structure according to the image data.

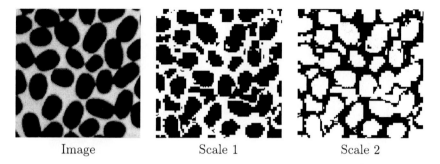

Image   Scale 1   Scale 2

Figure 2. Example texture from the Brodatz album with beans on a homogeneous background. The images in the middle and right show in white the areas with texture at the corresponding dyadic scale. Texture has been found at the scales 1 and 2 only. The scale selection algorithm determines the sharp borders as scale 1 texture and the patches of homogeneous foreground and background as textural objects at scale 2.

2.4 Estimation of the "characteristic" scale

The recursive fine-to-coarse and coarse-to-fine steps are iterated until the MAP probability (3) reaches a maximum. From the MAP configuration we deduce the "characteristic" scale by selecting for each branch of the pyramid the scale with the highest transition variance θ_p^2. This is the scale where the parent differs at most from its children, since the transition variance is a measure of the dissimilarity of children and its parent. In other words, at that scale the amount of information that the parent encodes about its children is minimal. Eq. (13) reflects this: A big transition variance means a small influence of the parent on the MAP-state of the child. An RV of the MSRF that has the maximum transition variance on a branch is marked as a texture object. The texture object is given by a the scale value of the RV and the region covered by all of its children.

2.5 Properties of the algorithm

An important feature of the algorithm is its hierarchical structure. This allows a fast scale sequential optimization of the MSRF. An extremum of the probability is usually reached within a few iterations. Further, the algorithm differs clearly from any linear filtering approach. Though an RV can be considered as a weighted average of its children, the set of children from which the average is taken is adapted to the data. It is not restricted to a quadratic region as in usual filtering. Additionally no artificial threshold is involved in

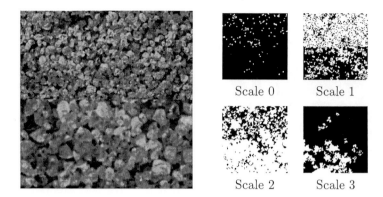

Scale 0   Scale 1

Scale 2   Scale 3

Figure 3. Analysis of an image containing grainy sand recorded at two scales. The scale of the texture does not match exactly with a dyadic scale. The upper half gives mainly evidence for texture at scale 1 and scale 2, while the lower half gives most evidence for texture at scale 2 and scale 3.

the scale selection algorithm. Since the selection involves only a maximization of the transition variance —which can be interpreted as a "generalized" local gray level variance— it is independent of the contrast and absolute brightness of the image.

3   Applications

3.1   Brodatz images

The algorithm is suitable for any kind of gray level images. First we give some results on images with homogeneous textures taken from the Brodatz album [12]. In the examples, we show the image, and the regions at the dyadic scales where texture has been found. The regions are marked in white and correspond to the ensemble of texture objects that have been found at that scale. Texture objects at the same scale are pairwise non-overlapping. However a fine scale texture may always be a part of a coarse scale texture. So that texture objects from different scales may overlap.

In Fig. 2 we show an example from the Brodatz texture album. It contains textures at only two scales: Texture at scale 1 corresponds to the sharp borders and texture at scale 2 corresponds to the homogeneous foreground and background patches. The second example in Fig. 3 is a composition of two images with grainy sand at two scales. The image structures are irregular and can not be clearly assigned to a dyadic scale. However it can be seen that

 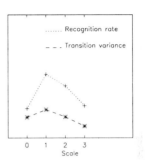

Figure 4. The image is an example of the MeasTex image database and shows a pebble path texture. On the right we plot the average variance at the different scales of the MSRF model. The maximum is at scale 1 at this scale we expect the most stringent texture. The second curve shows the rate of correct recognition of the texture using a MRF model. The recognition rate is maximal if the features are computed at the characteristic scale.

the lower half contains a texture at twice the resolution as the upper half.

3.2 Classification at the "characteristic" scale

Using publicly available images from the MeasTex image database [13] we have evaluated the performance of the scale selection scheme in combination with a Markov random field texture model [3]. The set of images contains various photographs of natural textures like asphalt, grass and different types of gravel and rocks. We have selected thirty different images as a set of reference textures and evaluated the classifications of new images. When the Markov random field model with a fixed kernel size has been applied to the images at the original scale we obtained an average rate of correct classification of 48%. In a second run we computed first the "characteristic" scale according to the MSRF model. Then we scaled the images to that scale and performed the classification with the MRF texture model. The overall percentage of correct classification increased to 53%. Fig. 4 gives an example texture of the MeasTex image set. On the right side we plot the average variance of the transition PDF of the MSRF. Its maximum indicates the "characteristic" scale. At this scale the rate of correct recognition peaks also.

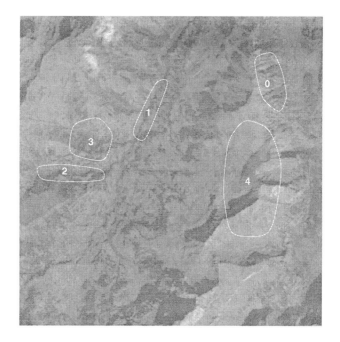

Figure 5. Scale selection on a Landsat TM scene. The scene contains different regions with textures at different scales. The "characteristic" scales of the delineated regions are printed in the image.

3.3 Scale Detection in Remote-sensing Data

The third example, Fig. 5, is a scenario of content based query in our remote-sensing database [8]. The database has precomputed signal-oriented content indices for all images. A user can define cover-types in an example image and search for this cover-type in the database. With the precomputed MSRF parameters the system can determine for each region the "characteristic" scale. In a subsequent database query the system will use the texture indices of this scale to find relevant images.

The example image is a taken from a Landsat image of a mountainous area in Switzerland. Image textures are due to the clouds, forested areas and geological drainage structures. These textures occur at different scales and give the different responses for the scale selection. The numbers in the delineated regions indicate the "characteristic" scale.

4 Conclusion

We have presented an algorithm for scale selection. This is an important issue in image texture analysis. Scale selection can be utilized as a preprocessing step before the actual texture analysis. Through the hierarchical structure it is fast and the computing time negligible as compared to running a more exhaustive texture model. The algorithm returns texture objects that consist of a scale number and a region. These can be used as masks for other texture models.

The benefits are twofold. First, by using the texture objects we can limit the further processing to those regions and scales where texture is expected to be found. This reduces the computing time. Second, it reduces the number of features to be used and therefore eases the task of classification.

In the current version, the algorithm has been implemented for scalar gray levels, correspondingly the RV are also scalar. However the theory and the algorithm can be extended to higher dimensions so that color images or other multi-dimensional spatial data can be processed.

Appendix

For the computation of the MAP distributions we need some properties of the Gaussian PDF. A Gaussian PDF with mean μ and variance σ is given by

$$\mathcal{N}\left(x - \mu, \sigma^2\right) = \frac{1}{\sqrt{2\pi}\,\sigma} e^{-\frac{1}{2}\left(\frac{x-\mu}{\sigma}\right)^2}. \tag{14}$$

From this we can directly derive

$$\mathcal{N}\left(x - \mu, \sigma^2\right) = \mathcal{N}\left(a(x - \mu), a^2\sigma^2\right). \tag{15}$$

The product of two Gaussians is proportional to a Gaussian

$$\mathcal{N}\left(x - \mu_1, \sigma_1^2\right) \cdot \mathcal{N}\left(x - \mu_2, \sigma_2^2\right) \propto$$
$$\mathcal{N}\left(x - \mu_1 \frac{\sigma_2^2}{\sigma_1^2 + \sigma_2^2} - \mu_2 \frac{\sigma_1^2}{\sigma_1^2 + \sigma_2^2}, \frac{\sigma_1^2 \sigma_2^2}{\sigma_1^2 + \sigma_2^2}\right) \tag{16}$$

with an averaged mean value and a reduced variance. Also for the convolution of two Gaussians we obtain a Gaussian

$$\sum_x \mathcal{N}\left(x - \mu_1, \sigma_1^2\right) \mathcal{N}\left(y - x - \mu_2, \sigma_2^2\right) = \mathcal{N}\left(y - (\mu_1 + \mu_2), \sigma_1^2 + \sigma_2^2\right). \tag{17}$$

This is the distribution of an RV that is the sum of two Gaussian RVs.

References

1. T. Randen and J. Husoy. Filtering for texture classification: A comparative study. *IEEE Trans. on Pattern Analysis and Machine Intelligence*, 21(4):291–309, 1999.
2. S. Krishnamachari and R. Chellappa. Multiresolution Gauss-Markov random field models for texture segmentation. *IEEE Trans. on Image Processing*, 6:251–267, 1997.
3. M. Schröder, H. Rehrauer, K. Seidel, and M. Datcu. Spatial information retrieval from remote sensing images—Part II: Gibbs Markov random fields. *IEEE Trans. on Geoscience and Remote Sensing*, 36(5):1446–1455, 1998.
4. J. Mao and A. Jain. Texture classification and segmentation using multiresolution simultaneous autoregressive models. *Pattern Recognition*, 25(2):173–188, 1992.
5. M. R. Luettgen, W. C. Karl, A. S. Willsky, and R. R. Tenney. Multiscale representations of Markov random fields. *IEEE Trans. on Signal Processing*, 41(12):3377–3396, 1993.
6. T. Lindeberg. Feature detection with automatic scale selection. *Int. J. of Computer Vision*, 30(2):77–116, 1998.
7. T. Lindeberg. *Scale-Space Theory in Computer Vision*. Kluwer, 1994.
8. H. Rehrauer and M. Schröder. Multi-mission demonstrator for content-based queries in remote sensing data (MMDEMO). http://www.vision.ee.ethz.ch/~rsia/, 1999.
9. M. Ramoni and P. Sebastiani. Bayesian methods for intelligent data analysis. Technical report, Knowledge Media Institute, http://kmi.open.ac.uk/people/marco, 1998.
10. Ch. A. Bouman and M. Shapiro. A multiscale random field model for Bayesian image segmentation. *IEEE Trans. on Image Processing*, 3(2):162–177, 1994.
11. H. Rehrauer, K. Seidel, and M. Datcu. Bayesian image segmentation using a dynamic pyramidal structure. In W. Linden, V. Dose, R. Fischer, and R. Preuss, editors, *Maximum Entropy and Bayesian Methods*, Fundamental Theories of Physics, pages 115–122, 1998.
12. P. Brodatz. *A Photographic Album for Artists and Designers*. Dover, New York, 1966.
13. G. Smith. MeasTex Image Texture Database and Test Suite. http://www.cssip.elec.uq.edu.au/~guy/meastex/meastex.html, 1997.

TEXTURE SEGMENTATION BASED ON THE UNIFORMITY TESTING AND NEURAL NETWORKS POSTPROCESSING

KATARZYNA MOŚCIŃSKA AND GRZEGORZ TYMA

Institute of Electronics, Silesian University of Technology, Akademicka 16, 44-101 Gliwice, Poland

E-mail: moscinsk@polsl.gliwice.pl

Textured images are often represented by stochastic models like Markov Random Fields (MRF). Usually, segmentation of images modelled by MRF is performed by the minimization of energy function during a relaxation procedure. This approach, however usually successful, is also computationally prohibitive.The alternative is to discriminate textures according to the MRF parameters considered as feature vectors of particular image classes. We model the pixel intensity by an MRF, but instead of energetic approach we propose the two-stage segmentation algorithm based on region splitting methods and neural networks concepts. During the first stage the rough segmentation on the basis of the estimated Gaussian Markov Random Field (GMRF) parameters is performed. In many real-life problems the obtained precision may be quite satisfactory. Optionally, the postprocessing stage in order to obtain more precise segmentation can be considered. In the paper the authors propose the implementation of neural networks for that task.

1 Introduction

Image segmentation belongs to the most challenging problems in computer vision. Segmentation becomes more complicated in case of textured images, i.e. images with rapid changes of pixel intensities over small distances - for such images the majority of the methods based on the detection of discontinuities are useless. When the textures are represented by feature vectors, some "classical" methods, like region splitting or clustering algorithms can be adopted for segmentation task. The alternative is the application of the spatial interaction models, like Markov Random Fields. Utilization of probabilistic models provides more sophisticated tools for image description as well as segmentation.

Spatial interaction models have been applied for modelling texture intensity, region geometry or boundary process (e.g. by Chellappa et al. [2], Cohen and Cooper [4], Geman and Geman [5], Manjunath and Chellappa [8]). Usually, application of MRF models leads to probabilistic segmentation performed by the maximization of the global *a posteriori* probability of pixel labels (MAP), conditioned by the class densities and *a priori* knowledge about the so called "region geometry". In case of textured images the hierarchic MRF models become extremely complicated, and the global energy function that should be minimized cannot be decomposed into local energy terms, which is necessary in order to perform iterative segmentation based on local computations. In such case some alleviation of the constraints imposed on the global energy function must be introduced, and in such case only local maximum of the posterior density can be obtained.

As the MRF models have been proved to be the satisfactory means of texture representation, some alternative approaches to the MAP concept can be considered. Chellappa and Chatterjee [3] succeeded in classification of texture samples based on features computed from GMRF parameters. Panjwani and Healey [11] propose multistage segmentation of color texture images based on region splitting methods, with the final stage of segmentation based on the maximization of the pseudolikelihood function, introduced by Silverman and Cooper [12]. Mościńska [9,10] proposed the two stage segmentation, with the first stage based on the clustering techniques, and the fine segmentation performed by the minimization of the energy function, but only in the limited area of the picture.

In many image processing applications the computation time of image segmentation is more crucial than the segmentation precision. Mościńska [10] proposed the segmentation method based on region splitting and clustering algorithms. The result of the proposed method is the labelling of the *block* of pixels, which size is limited by the number of points required for reliable estimation of the GMRF parameters. In the paper we present the modification of the method introduced in Mościńska [10], and propose the postprocessing stage that leads to the fine segmentation. The postprocessing is performed by the backpropagation network, which is applied in order to label pixels in the boundary area. Some other methods of the postprocessing, like minimization of the energy function in the limited area of the picture, can also be considered for that purpose.

2 Image Modelling with Markov Random Fields Models

A collection of random variables $\boldsymbol{X} = X_s, s \in S$ is an MRF if:

$$P(X_s = x_s | X_t = x_t; t \neq s) = P(X_s = x_s | X_t = x_t; t \in \eta_s), \qquad (1)$$

where $S = s_1, s_2, ..., s_N$ is the set of sites in the $M \times M = N$ point lattice, and η_s, called neigborhood, is a subset of S.

MRF representation is computationaly tractable due to Hammersley – Clifford theorem, see Besag [1], which establishes the equivalence between the MRF and the Gibbs distribution: $\boldsymbol{X}$ is a MRF $\Leftrightarrow P(\boldsymbol{X} = \boldsymbol{x}) =$

$\frac{1}{Z} \exp \{-U(\boldsymbol{x})/T\}$, where T is a scaling parameter, and Z is a normalizing constant.

An important class of MRFs are Gaussian Markov Random Fields (GMRF). When the Markov property (1) is satisfied, and the local probability density functions $p(x_s)$ are gaussian, then the following holds (see Woods [13]):

$$x_s = \mu_s + \sum_{t \in \eta_s} \beta_{st}(x_t - \mu_t) + e_s, \qquad (2)$$

where μ_s is the mean value of the field, $\{\beta_{st}\}$ are the parameters of the model, whereas e_s denotes the stationary zero-mean gaussian noise, with the following autocorrelation matrix:

$$\mathrm{E}\,[e_s e_t] = \begin{cases} -\beta_{st}\sigma^2 & \text{for } t \in \eta_s, \\ \sigma^2 & \text{for } t = s, \\ 0 & \text{otherwise} \end{cases} \qquad (3)$$

The estimation of the Gaussian Markov Random Field (GMRF) parameters can be performed as follows (see Kashyap and Chellappa [7]):

$$\hat{\beta} = \left[\sum_{x_i \in S^I} \boldsymbol{x}_{\eta_i} \boldsymbol{x}_{\eta_i}^T \right]^{-1} \left[\sum_{x_i \in S^I} \boldsymbol{x}_{\eta_i} x_i \right], \qquad (4)$$

$$\hat{\sigma}^2 = \frac{1}{n} \sum_{x_i \in S^I} \left(x_i - \beta^T \boldsymbol{x}_{\eta_i} \right)^2, \qquad (5)$$

where the summation extends over the non-boundary sites S^I of the lattice S, and n denotes the number of sites considered.

3 Division of Nonuniform Regions (DNR) Method

The proposed DNR method can be considered as the "region–splitting" algorithm. The image is iteratively partitioned into a number of square regions according to the uniformity criterion, which is based on the values of the GMRF parameters (4,5). The procedure starts with the largest square — the whole image — and proceeds until all the regions are uniform, or become too small to be further split (i.e. uniformity criterion cannot be evaluated). The proposed DNR algorithm was designed in order to perform the rough segmentation of textured images, which means that the result of the procedure is the labelling of a *block* of pixels, instead of a *single* pixel. We assume that the segmentation is unsupervised, i.e. the GMRF parameters of the various parts (classes) of the image are unknown. The maximum number of classes N_K must be limited in advance.

The uniformity criterion is based on the values of the GMRF parameters (4,5), evaluated in a square as well as its four sub-squares. Let us substitute β_j for β_{st} in (2) for clarity reasons. The square uniformity is tested according to the evaluated value of the uniformity parameter D_β:

$$D_\beta = \max_m \sum_j \left(\beta_j^i - \beta_j^m \right)^2 \qquad (6)$$

where β_j^i and β_j^m denote the jth GMRF parameter computed for the whole square i and its four subsquares, respectively, and m is the index of subsquares, $m = 1, ..., 4$. The square is considered uniform when D_β is lower than the predefined threshold value ϵ^β. The value of ϵ^β is heuristic and depends mostly on the maximum number of texture classes N_K present in the analysed image.

When the analysed square i is found uniform, the *class matching indicators* $(C_{i,k})$ for all currently defined classes $l_k = 1, ..., N_K$ are evaluated in the following way:

$$C_{i,k} = \frac{\left\| \beta^i - \beta^k \right\|}{\left\| \beta^i \right\|} + \rho \frac{\left| \sigma^i - \sigma^k \right|}{\sigma^i}, \qquad (7)$$

where β^i, σ^i, β^k, σ^k are the GMRF parameters of the square i and the class k, respectively, and ρ is a weighing multiplier. If the first uniform square is considered, or the minimum value of all the $C_{i,k}$ exceeds the predefined threshold value ϵ^d, the new class is defined, or the existing class parameters are redefined.

The final result of the DNR procedure are:

- the GMRF parameters of all the classes N_K present in the analysed image,

- labelling all the image pixels with a label corresponding to one of the classes l_k.

The most original part of the DNR algorithm is the redefinition of the texture classes, described in details in Mościńska [10].

The performance of the DNR approach has been tested on many real life as well as synthetic textures, and the majority of the obtained results was very promising.

The GMRF parameters cannot be reliably evaluated, when the number of pixels n considered for estimation is lower than twice the number of the

GMRF parameters (see Panjwani [11]). The smallest side of a square utilized in the DNR procedure is $N_{P\,min} = 8$ pixels. Consequently, the evaluated texture boundary is rather "sharp". If the problem requires more precise evaluation of the border line, the postprocessing stage must be applied. The authors propose the implementation of neural network for that task. It should be emphasised, however, that the segmentation becomes much more complicated and time consuming, which is a typical trade-off in image segmentation tasks.

4 Refinement of the Pixel Labelling in the Boundary Areas Performed with Neural Networks

If the "block-labelling" accuracy is not satisfactory, the post-processing segmentation stage should be considered. The authors propose the application of the backpropagation neural network (see Hecht-Nielsen [6]) for the final labelling of pixels in the boundary areas. Below, the idea of neural relabelling will be described, with the main stress laid on the problem of choosing the boundary area, and the evaluation of the input signal for the network.

Definition of the boundary area

Various options for choosing the boundary area can be considered. Firstly, either only the part, or the whole border should be verified. Secondly, the "width" of the boundary area may vary, thus influencing the obtained precision of boundary extraction. Moreover, the distance between the pixels considered for relabelling can be modified, which also results in various precision levels obtained in the second stage. One possible approach for choosing the boundary area is to consider all the points, that fulfilz the following condition: let S_L denotes a square of size $N_L \times N_L$ points, around a pixel i, placed in the middle of the square. If all the labels l_i of the pixels belonging to the square are the same, than the central pixel i will not be considered for relabelling. Otherwise, the central pixel will become the subject of the boundary refinement. The proposed size N_L should be at least as big as the size of the smallest block of pixels considered for the GMRF parameters estimation.

Definition of the input signal for a neural network.

Our aim is to classify the points according to the estimated GMRF parameters. In the boundary areas pixels of more than one class have been utilized for the GMRF parameters estimation, so those vectors of parameters do not represent properly a class. The input signal for the neural network should be chosen so that this effect could be somehow compensated. We propose the following evaluation of the input signal for the neural network: each pixel i is identified with a number N_N of partially overlapping squares, that are used for the GMRF parameters estimation. The estimated parameters $\{\boldsymbol{\beta}^n\}, n = 1...N_N$, arranged as one vector, constitute the input signal for the neural network. Typical numbers of N_N are of the range 5 to 9 squares, the size of the squares N_β is 16 by 16 pixels, and the overlap is between one third and one fourth of the square size in each dimension. Therefore, for the 5 overlapping squares, and the 10-element GMRF vector $\boldsymbol{\beta}^n$, there is a 50-elements input signal for the network. Optionally, two additional values, referring to the standard deviation σ and mean value μ (2, 3) can be included in the input signal. The network training is performed as follows: Firstly, some equally spaced points of the image are extracted. Typically, 100 to 1000 points can be considered. For each point the input signal for the network is evaluated as stated above. The three-layer backpropagation neural network requires usually not more than 50 iterations (full sweeps) for proper classification of input signals.

The relabelling of the pixels in the boundary area is performed according to the neural network classification (testing phase). For each pixel considered the input signal must be evaluated in the same manner as for the training samples. The pixels are relabelled according to the network output. The evaluation of the input signal is relatively fast, due to the linear procedures for the GMRF parameter estimation (see Kashyap and Chellappa [7]).

The described procedure is definitely much more time consuming than the first stage of image processing, leading to the rough segmentation. As the obtained results of the second stage are very satisfactory, the postprocessing stage can be suggested for applications where the precision of segmentation is of the greatest importance. This refers in particular to the problems which require processing of the great number of images of similar class.

5   Segmentation Results

The DNR algorithm together with the NN - postprocessing stage has been tested on many textured images, with varying parameters like the order of the GMRF model, the threshold values of the parameters applied for the uniformity testing as well as for the class matching. The results of segmentation are quite good even for typical threshold values ϵ^β and ϵ^d, and are very satisfactory when the threshold parameter can be tuned during experiments, i.e.

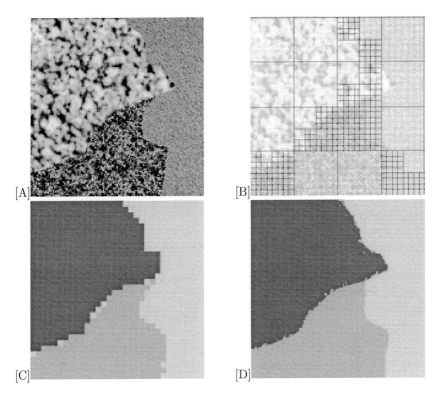

Figure 1. Consecutive phases of textured image segmentation.

the set of pictures of similar nature is available.

Below, typical segmentation results will be presented. The exemplary image, which was generated in the synthetic manner, consists of three various textured regions. Pixel intensity was modelled with the third order GMRF which corresponds to six parameters β_j. The first stage of segmentation (DNR procedure) was performed with the following threshold values: $\epsilon^\beta = 0.02$, $\epsilon^d = 0.1$, $\rho = 0.3$. The minimum side of the square used for the GMRF parameters estimation is $N_{P\min} = 8$.

Fig. 1A presents the image to be segmented. The successive region divisions according to the nonuniformity of texture performed during the DNR stage are illustrated by Fig. 1B. The final result of the DNR stage is presented in Fig. 1C. The obtained rough segmentation is quite good for the image considered, as well as for the majority of other images that were processed.

After completing the first stage of segmentation, the neural network post-processing was performed. The following neural network was used: three-layer backpropagation network, with 40 neurons in the input and hidden layers, and 3 neurons in the output layer (see previous section). The network was trained with 120 input vectors, selected so that both uniform and nonuniform regions were represented. After 57 iterations the network training was completed - the ratio of proper classification for the training set was 100%. Two experiments were carried out, with testing vectors chosen from either uniform, or nonuniform parts of the image. 93% of the uniform samples were classified correctly, whereas for the set referring to the nonuniform regions the obtained classification accuracy was 85%. The refinement of the boundary labels obtained with the neural network is presented in Fig. 1D. Similar ratios have been obtained in other experiments.

According to the rule of thumb, that the number of training vectors should be at least ten times of the number of neurons, the proposed training set is to small for the particular network. However, during other experiments the number of training patters was increased up to 1000, which is quite proper for such a network. When the problem becomes more complicated, the number of input patterns should be definitely much larger than in the described experiment.

6 Conclusions

In the paper the concept of two-stage segmentation of textured images has been presented. The authors proposed simple and successful algorithm for rough segmentation of textured images. Image pixel intensity is modelled with the Gaussian Markov Random Field. The GMRF parameters are applied for image uniformity testing. The segmentation algorithm is unsupervised, i.e. the GMRF parameters of various classes are assumed to be unknown in advance. The DNR algorithm is robust to the values of the thresholding parameters. The effectiveness of the algorithm results from the block-processing during the segmentation.

The refinement of the pixel labelling in the boundary areas can be performed in many ways. The authors were successful with applying the back-propagation neural networks for that task. The other approach to be considered is the minimization of the global energy function in the limited area of the picture.

References

1. J. Besag, "Spatial interaction and the statistical analysis of lattice systems (with discussion)", *J. Royal Statist. Soc.* B **36**, 192 (1974), 192–326.
2. R. Chellappa, B. S. Manjunath and T. Simchony, "Texture segmentation with neural networks", *Texture segmentation with neural networks* in *Neural networks for signal processing*, ed. B. Kosko (Prentice Hall, New York, 1992), 37–61.
3. R. Chellappa and S. Chatterjee, "Classification of textures using Gaussian Markov Random Fields", *IEEE Trans. Acoust. Speech Signal Process* **33**, 959 (1985), 959–963.
4. F. Cohen and D. Cooper, "Simple Parallel Hierarchical and Relaxation Algorithms for Segmenting Noncausal Markovian Random Fields", *IEEE Trans. Pattern Anal. Machine Intell.* **9**, 195 (1987), 195–219.
5. S. Geman and D. Geman, "Stochastic relaxation, Gibbs distributions, and the Bayesian restoration of images", *IEEE Trans. Pattern Anal. Machine Intell.* **6**, 721 (1984), 721–741.
6. R. Hecht-Nielsen, *Neurocomputing* (Addison-Wesley, 1989).
7. R. Kashyap and R. Chellappa, "Estimation and Choice of Neighbors in Spatial-Interaction Models of Images", *IEEE Trans. on Information Theory* **29**, 60 (1983), 60–72.
8. B.S. Manjunath and R. Chellappa, "Unsupervised Texture Segmentation Using Markov Random Field models", *IEEE Trans. Pattern Anal. Machine Intell.* **13**, 478 (1991), 478–482.
9. K. Mościńska, "Markov Random Field Models for Supervised and Unsupervised Segmentation of Texture Images", *Proceedings of Workshop on Design Methodologies for Signal Processing* **1**, 92 (1996), 192–197.
10. K. Mościńska, *Metody segmentacji obrazów teksturowych z wykorzystaniem wielowymiarowych modeli Markowa* (in Polish), (Ph.D. thesis, Wydział Automatyki, Elektroniki i Informatyki, Politechnika Śląska, Gliwice, 1998).
11. D. K. Panjwani and G. Healey, "Markov Random Field Models for Unsupervised Segmentation of Textured Color Images", *IEEE Trans. Pattern Anal. Machine Intell.* **17**, 939 (1995), 939–954.
12. J. Silverman and D. Cooper, "Bayesian Clustering for Unsupervised Estimation of Surface and Texture Models", *IEEE Trans. Pattern Anal. Machine Intell.* **10**, 481 (1988), 481–495.
13. J.W. Woods, "Two-Dimensional Discrete Markovian Random Fields", *IEEE Transactions on Information Theory* **18**, 232 (1972), 232–240.

MULTI-RESOLUTION CLUSTERING OF TEXTURE IMAGES

SEBASTIANO BATTIATO AND GIOVANNI GALLO

Dipartimento di Matematica, Università di Catania, Viale A. Doria 6, 95125, Catania, Italy.

E-mail: {battiato, gallo}@dipmat.unict.it

The focus of this paper is mainly on texture synthesis rather than analysis. We describe a new method for analysis/synthesis of textures using a non-parametric multi-resolution approach. In the analysis step the new technique clusters together structural features with the same visual appearance from an input texture using a standard pyramid-based decomposition. The synthesis is obtained through a sampling procedure constraining the distribution of the spatial characteristics at lower resolution. This is realized through a new data structure called *frequency tree* that implicitly describes the texture itself. Experimental results show the effectiveness of such approach: it is capable to reproduce efficiently the generative stochastic process of a wide class of real texture images. The proposed method achieves a greater computational efficiency than other approach known in the literature.

1 Introduction

Computer Graphics is interested in textures because their use can greatly enhance the sense of realism of a polygonal scene. Goal of the texture synthesis is to create a texture which is at the same time, random and perceptually not distinguishable from the original. This task, that may look at first contradictory, may be achieved in several ways. Statistical regularities are good tools to model and understand the complex stochastic nature of basic textural elements: indeed qualitative statistical texture analysis occurs in the human visual system [1]. Techniques to learn and to reproduce the generative process of a texture, have been extensively investigated for their applications and for the insights that they can bring in understanding human vision.

More recently the idea of using multi-resolution analysis and synthesis for pattern and textures has been investigated by many [6,10,17,18,19], but a practical and efficient way to reproduce faithfully every natural texture acquired from the physical/natural world is yet to be found. The new algorithm proposed in this paper, similarly to De Bonet [6], uses a pyramid-based technique in order to analyze the details of the textures in input. What we try to do differently is to use cluster analysis at several resolution levels to speed up by an important factor the synthesis of a texture. In this way we are able to compact together the regions with similar structural characteristics with respect to a well-defined feature detector. Similar ideas have been discussed in a very different context by Lepsoy and Oien [12] and Ramamurthi and Gersho [14]: in the search for domain-range affinity in a picture to achieve fractal compression they suggest, indeed, to cluster together similar ranges in order to speed up computation.

The synthesis of new textures is obtained sampling from the distribution built in the analysis phase. Such a distribution is constrained by the relative history of the frequencies with respect to the various clusters at each level (see below for more details). The main advance offered by this approach with respect to previous known methods is a better computational efficiency at synthesis phase together with the ability to reproduce an exhaustive set of real textures. Experimental results show that the proposed algorithm works up to 5 times faster than the algorithm in [6].

The present paper is arranged as follows. The next section reviews some previous results in the literature. Section 3 describes the details of our approach. Results are reported and discussed in Section 4 and, finally, conclusions and directions for future research are sketched in Section 5.

2   Texture Model and Synthesis

Analysis and synthesis of textured images is generally restated as a statistical inference problem. According to this approach all the relevant information about a texture are obtained filtering the input pattern with a suitable linear or non-linear filter bank. The most updated statistical theory for texture modeling can be found in [17,18,19] where filtering theory, information theoretical arguments and Markov Random Field [5] are combined together. Equally important in pattern synthesis is the multi-resolution approach: almost all recent studies regarding texture modeling take this approach with the standard Laplacian and Gaussian pyramid decomposition [3,13,15]. Heeger and Bergen pioneered this methodology in 1995. They propose an iterative procedure with an internal equalization of the relative histograms. Their algorithm synthesizes textures using first order statistics of the distribution of image energy as a function of position, scale, frequency and orientation. Although powerful this approach is not able to reproduce complex and/or highly stochastic textures. But is it an explicit, full statistical model of a texture necessary in order to reproduce it, at least at perceptual level? A negative answer to this question, hence a good news for computer graphics, comes from some recent results.

In 1997, De Bonet has proposed an effective and qualitatively more expressive sampling methodology; he introduces a multi-resolution sampling procedure in which each particular RGB value of the pixels is constrained, at every level of the Laplacian pyramid, by its *history* with respect to the lower resolution levels. The data structure used by De Bonet to keep track of this history is called *parent vector* of a pixel. The *parent vector* of a pixel hence, is a structure whose components are the local response for each feature at every lower resolution. To capture the effective features of a particular texture each level of the Gaussian pyramid is convoluted with a filter bank containing edge and line detection operators. The underlying hypothesis of this sampling methodology is that, in texture images, some features are more recognizable at certain resolutions than other. The value of each pixel is successively sampled from a set containing all the pixel values whose parent structure is close with respect to a given measure of similarity. This algorithm models well a large set of real textures but it is computationally expensive. One of its bottlenecks is the sampling step: classes of pixels with similar parent structures are not explicitly available and sampling is done, at each step, from the whole pixel population. Several tries may be needed until a sufficiently good sample is found. We propose at this regard two major improvements over De Bonet's work. First of all we are able to obtain a dramatic speed up of the algorithm implementing, together with few of the heuristic proposed by De Bonet himself, the novel idea of reducing the sampling space through a suitable clustering at each level of the resolution pyramid. The second significant result comes as a by-product of the clustering heuristic: we obtain an *implicit statistical model* of the input texture. This model (called *frequency tree*) is described as a tree data structure that contains information about the co-occurrence of some features at the different resolution levels. It is important to observe that in our approach, the *frequency tree* has to be computed only once for an input texture. Successive generation of similar textures does not require the repetition of the relatively costly clustering and analysis procedure. The interest of the *frequency tree* goes beyond the synthesis of a pattern: we claim that they can be used as statistical signatures of a texture and hence can be of great help in pattern recognition and in image database retrieval.

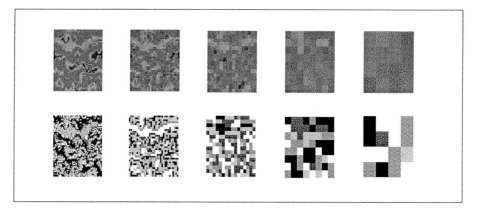

Figure 1. A standard Gaussian-pyramid and its corresponding clustering

3   Our Approach

We proceed in two distinct phases. First the input image is analyzed with respect to its structural components at different resolutions. On the basis of the information collected, it is possible to sample the synthesized texture. The details of our technique are reported below.

3.1   Analysis phase

The input texture I is decomposed following a standard pyramid-based procedure. This operation allows to detect some features of the texture under observation, at different levels of resolution. Denote with $G_0 = I$, G_1, ... , G_N and with L_1, ... , L_{N-1} respectively the corresponding octave-spaces of the Gaussian pyramid and of the Laplacian pyramid.

Each Gaussian octave G_i is in turn convoluted with a set of edge and line detection filters. Texture features are the output of such filters. In particular, following the original De Bonet's proposal, in our experiments, we use 3x3 Sobel filters and binomial filters.

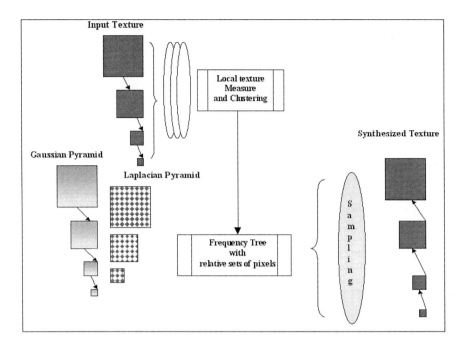

Figure 2. A schematic description, along the line of [6] of our approach.

Using the information obtained from such convolutions, each Gaussian octave is clustered. *Clustering* is a process to partition a given set of pixels in a set of *k* smaller subgroups, by the use of a resemblance or difference measure. As a difference measure we have adopted, in the experiments, a simple isotropic euclidean distance in the feature space. Better results could be found, at higher computational cost, using perceptually more significant difference measures.

Clustering is an essential tool for data analysis and has taken a central role also in vision algorithms [4]. Many techniques have been developed for clustering data: c-means clustering, adaptive vector quantization (AVQ), and the self-organizing maps (SOM) [4,9,11]. In our experiments, for sake of efficiency, we adopted a simple hard c-mean clustering procedure.

Figure 1 shows in the lower part, the partition obtained at the successive Gaussian octaves of the given input texture, with different gray tones for each cluster. The number of clusters to consider is an important parameter for the quality of final results. We found experimentally that, at high and middle resolution, five clusters are generally a good choice. At lower resolution a smaller number of cluster could be safely used, however, for sake of an homogeneous implementation we adopted five clusters for every level without noticeable losses in quality and efficiency. Denote with $\mathbf{P}_{ij}$, $i=0, ..., N-1$, $j=1, ... , k_i$ the j-th cluster obtained at the i-th resolution level. Hence at level i we have k_i different clusters. The knowledge of $\mathbf{P}_{ij}$ classes allows to generate an *history* of each pixel and its immediate neighbors along the various pyramid levels. In particular, we compute the relative frequencies of each cluster at level i with respect to the clusters at the lower resolution level $i+1$. The information gathered in this way is organized in a tree summarizing the statistical properties of the pixel population. We refer to this tree as the *frequency tree* of the input texture. The tree has height equal to the number of pyramid levels, while the numbers of possible paths is equal to k_1 x k_2 x .. x k_{N-1} . Each leaf corresponds to a set of pixels: all the pixels in the same leaf share the same *history* at different resolutions.

3.2 Synthesis phase

The synthesis of a new texture relies on an explicitly computed statistical model i.e. the frequency tree built in the analysis phase. The procedure goes as sketched below.

Phase 0
Reconstruction of lowest resolution level.
Phase 1
For every successive level i:
Assign every pixel at this level to one of the clusters $P_{i1}, ... P_{iki}$ respecting relative frequencies using *frequency tree*. In this way every pixels has, up to the i-th level, a complete history. Observe that the pixels in a 2x2 square have a common history up to the $(i-1)$-th level. It is at this step that they may stray down different paths of the *frequency tree*. Every 2x2 square, hence, can be characterized by a common history, up to level $(i-1)$, for its four pixels, and by the four labels of the cluster assigned to each pixel at the i-th level. Let $(h, j_1, j_2, j_3, j_4)=h_Q$ denote the history of the square Q.
For each 2x2 square Q at this level assign a 2x2 square of Laplacian triplets chosen from the 2x2 square of Laplacian triplets in the input texture, at the corresponding level, that are characterized by the same vector h_Q.
Phase 2
Collapse the pyramid into a unique new texture.

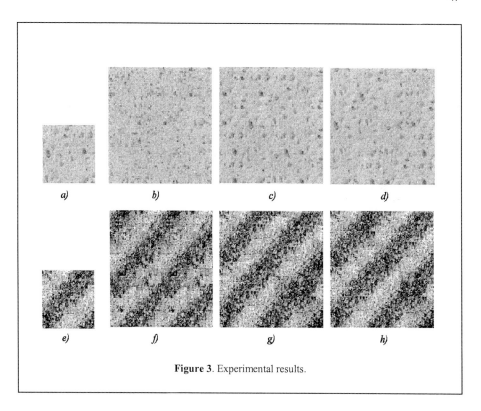

Figure 3. Experimental results.

The process is summarized in Fig. 2. For each location at each level we have to perform two simple constrained random samplings: one is to assign a pixel to a cluster, the other to obtain the corresponding quartet of Laplacian RGB values. For a 2^N x 2^N texture, where the analysis has been carried out at N resolution levels the proposed method requires $O(2^{2N})$ random sampling operations. This upper bound cannot be guaranteed in the De Bonet's procedure: there random sampling has to be performed at each level over the whole pixel population. This require to visit, for each location to be sampled, all the corresponding parents vectors relative to all pixels in the corresponding input-pyramid, until a suitable pixel value is found. The advantage of our approach is already evident in synthesizing a texture of the same dimension than the original. The difference in performance between the two method becomes greater if a larger than the original texture has to be synthesized as shown from the data reported in the next section.

4   Experiments and discussion

In this Section we report the results obtained. We have implemented the algorithm above and a version of De Bonet's algorithm that we have tried to optimize at best of our knowledge. The language used has been MatLab 5 on a Pentium II 350 Mhz, 64 Mb RAM platform. Using these homogeneous implementations we have processed several input patterns of 64x64 pixels. Our analysis of the pattern generally requires a longer time than De Bonet's but we go much faster in the synthesis phase. Moreover, texture images of arbitrary dimension can be generated once the *frequency tree* of an input texture has been computed and stored. Table 1 shows the average time obtained in our implementation for the two algorithms.

Table 1. Average time obtained with the three different approaches.

	Our Approach	De Bonet	Mixed
Analysis	*26"*	*4"*	*26"*
Synthesis of 64x64	*3"*	*140"*	*30"*
Synthesis of 128x128	*15"*	*550"*	*122"*

A typical texture reconstructed from Fig.3.a or Fig.3.e with our algorithm is compared with the reconstruction obtained with De Bonet's algorithm in Fig. 3.b/3.c and Fig 3.f/3.g. It is evident that the performance of our approach is very good, although a slight quality loss can be observed for example comparing Fig.3.b on 3.c. We have found that a better quality of reconstruction can be obtained taking a mixed approach: instead of randomly sampling from a cluster for the Laplacian RGB values, we look for the *best* values among those in the cluster. Here *best* means closest in the De Bonet's parent vector sense. Timing of this mixed approach are also reported in Table 1. Texture reconstructed with the mixed approach are reported in Fig.3.d and Fig.3.h. It is evident that they are of the same quality than the reconstruction in Fig.3.c and Fig.3.g. Other textures synthesized with the mixed approach are reported in Fig.4.

Crucial to the class of textures that can be *learned* with our multi-resolution approach are the filters applied to the input texture before clusterization. A blind mixture of them can guarantee, in general, only half successful results. This comes not as a surprise: Zhu and Mumford [17] have strongly stressed the need to include in the learning process also the discrimination of an information-theoretical optimized mixture of filters.

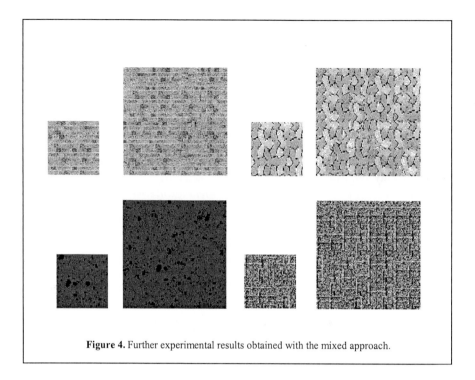

Figure 4. Further experimental results obtained with the mixed approach.

Less crucial appears, on the other hand, the clustering procedure adopted and the number of cluster chosen for every resolution level. All of the experiments have been realized partitioning pixel, at every resolution level, into four/five clusters. A higher number of clusters gave no improvements, while results obtained using fewer clusters are unsatisfactory.

5   Conclusions and Future Works

The paper has proposed an efficient multi-resolution clustered sampling procedure able to synthesize real texture images. Experimental results have been reported in order to prove the effectiveness of the new approach. The application of the ideas introduced here to discriminate texture images and measure their degree of similarity in real applications (e.g. SAR images) is object of our actual research. In particular it would be interesting to see how the proposed method would perform in texture classification/segmentation, in comparison to other mainstream paradigms.

References

1. J.R. Bergen, B. Julesz, Rapid Discrimination of Visual Patterns, IEEE Transactions on Systems Man and Cybernetics, 13:857-863, (1993).
2. P.Brodatz, Textures: A Photographic Album for Artists & Designers, Dover, New York, (1966).
3. P.J. Burt, E.H. Adelson, The Laplacian Pyramid as a Compact Image Code, IEEE Transactions on Communications, 31:532-540, (1983).
4. Z. Chi, H. Yan, T. Pham, Fuzzy Algorithm: With Applications to Image Processing and Pattern Recognition, World Scientific, 1996.
5. G.R. Cross, A.K. Jain, *Markov Random Field texture models*, IEEE, *PAMI*, 5, pp. 25-39, (1983).
6. J.S. De Bonet, Multiresolution Sampling Procedure for Analysis and Synthesis of Texture Images, In Computer Graphics, pp. 361-368, ACM SIGGRAPH, (1997).
7. J.S. De Bonet, *MIT Jeremy S. De Bonet's home page* - Demo of Texture Synthesis (`www.ai.mit.edu/~jsd/Research/TextureSynthesis`) (1997).
8. J.S. De Bonet, P. Viola, Texture Recognition Using a Non-parametric Multi-scale Statistical Model, In Proceedings IEEE Conf. on computer Vision and Pattern Recognition, (1998).
9. J. Dickerson, B. Kosko, Fuzzy Function Learning With Covariance Ellipsoids, In Proceedings IEEE International Conf. on Neural Network, Vol. III, pp. 1162-1167, San Francisco, USA, (1993).
10. D.J. Heeger, J.R. Bergen, Pyramid-Based Texture Analysis/Synthesis, In Computer Graphics, pp. 229-238, ACM SIGGRAPH, (1995).
11. T. Kohonen, The Self-Organizing Map, In Proceedings of IEEE, 78(9) pp.1464-1480, (1990).
12. S. Lepsoi, G.E. Oien, Fast Attractor Image Encoding by Adaptive Codebook Clustering, in Fractal Image Compression, Y. Fisher, Ed. Springer Verlag, pp. 177-197, (1994).
13. J.M. Ogden, E.H. Adelson, J.R. Bergen, P.J. Burt, Pyramid-Based Computer Graphics, *RCA Engineer* 30, pp. 4-15, (1985).
14. B. Ramamurthi, A. Gersho, Classified Vector Quantization of Images, *IEEE Trans. Comm.*, COM-34, pp. 1105-115, (1986).
15. E.P. Simoncelli, E.H. Adelson, *Subband Transform*, In *Subband Image Coding*, J.W Woods, Ed. Kluwer Academic Publishers, Norwell, MA, (1990).
16. E.P. Simoncelli, W.T. Freeman, E.H. Adelson, D.J. Heeger, Shiftable Multiscale Transform, IEEE Transactions on Information Theory 38, pp. 587-607, (1992).

17. S.C. Zhu, D. Mumford, Prior Learning and Gibbs Reaction-Diffusion, IEEE, *PAMI* Vol.18, no.11, pp. 1236-1250, Nov. (1997).
18. S.C. Zhu, Y.N. Wu, D. Mumford, Minimax Entropy Principle and Its Application to Texture Modeling, Neural Computation Vol.9, No.8, Nov. (1997).
19. S.C. Zhu, Y.N. Wu, D. Mumford, Filters, Random Fields And Maximum Entropy (FRAME*),* Int'l Journal of Computer Vision, 27(2) 1-20, March/April (1998).

A TEXTURE CLASSIFICATION SYSTEM
USING STATISTICAL AND SOFT-COMPUTING METHODS

ALEXANDER STOLPMANN

Fachhochschule Braunschweig/Wolfenbüttel, Fachbereich Informatik,
Salzdahlumer Straße 46/48, D-38302 Wolfenbüttel, Germany
E-mail: stolpmann@fh-wolfenbuettel.de

LAURENCE S. DOOLEY

Monash University, School of Computing and Information Technology,
Gippsland Campus, Churchill, Victoria 3842, Australia
E-mail: laurence.dooley@infotech.monash.edu.au

This paper describes the use of a complex modular image processing system for texture classification. An introduction into problems that arise when handling textures is given. Furthermore the modules of the proposed system are described, namely the filtering and statistical modules, the genetic algorithm module for automatic feature vector optimization and the classification modules using soft-computing methods.

1 Introduction

The real world does not supply the laboratory conditions that are necessary for the majority of the existing image processing systems. Therefore all those ill structured or coarse grained objects and especially objects without clear boundaries are a major problem in the field of object recognition. In some areas it is even problematical to speak of objects in the classical sense. One only has to think of a corn field, a lawn, ripples on water, clouds in the sky or leaves on a tree to comprehend the problems.

The aim of the research work of which this paper describes a part is to find a solution to the problem of classifying genuine texture, as texture represents the unstructuredness very well. Some alternative and completely new methods are being developed and tested. Furthermore existing approaches for sub-problems are included in the system. This system shall not be adapted for a special problem but shall be universal. Therefore it can be used for multiple tasks in many fields, e. g. medicine, remote sensing, machine vision, etc.

This paper describes modules used in the system, i. e. the filtering and statistical modules for feature extraction, the genetic algorithms for feature vector optimization and the fuzzy clustering and neural network modules for classification.

54

2 A Short Description of Texture

The word *texture*, which descends from the Latin word *texere* ("to weave"), is not uniquely defined, but rather described context dependently. The WEB-STER [21] definition closest to the use in image analysis is *similar qualities dependent on the nature and arrangement of the constituent particles of a substance.*

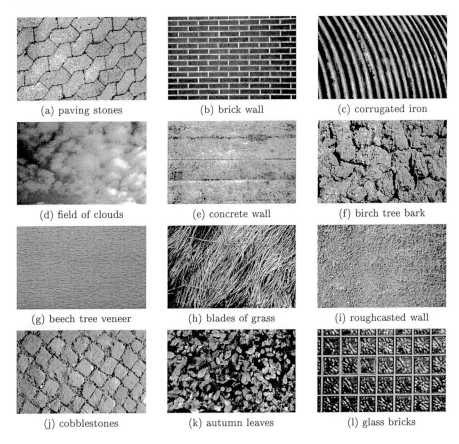

(a) paving stones   (b) brick wall   (c) corrugated iron

(d) field of clouds   (e) concrete wall   (f) birch tree bark

(g) beech tree veneer   (h) blades of grass   (i) roughcasted wall

(j) cobblestones   (k) autumn leaves   (l) glass bricks

Figure 1. Pictures of natural, half-natural and man-made texture.

In general it can be said that a texture describes the surface composition of an object. Texture can be divided into regular texture, composed of repeated texture primitives which are large against the pixel resolution and could be described in further detail (cf. fig. 1(a) – 1(c)), and statistical texture with texture primitives that near unity and have a random distribution (cf. fig. 1(d) – 1(i)). Very often texture is of a hierarchical kind where the macro texture is regular and the micro texture of statistically describable primitives (cf. fig. 1(j) – 1(l)).

2.1 Artificial and Genuine Texture

Two major groups of texture types exist[a], namely artificial and genuine texture.

Artificial texture is usually computer generated and thus well defined. Handling this kind of texture may result in the finding of parameters that describe the regularity instead of the texture itself.

Genuine texture on the other hand can only be found in our surroundings. To handle these photographs have to be taken and subsequently transferred into a computer readable format so that they can be handled for further investigation.

For testing the system only genuine texture is being used. This group can be subdivided into natural, half-natural and man-made texture, a classification introduced by the author in [17]. Textures cannot be assigned strictly but rather in a fuzzy way to a certain group.

2.2 Natural Texture

Natural textures are those that can be found in unspoilt nature, that means in areas untouched or unchanged by mankind. The figures 1(d), 1(f), 1(h) and 1(k) show some examples.

2.3 Man-Made Texture

In contrast to the natural textures some man-made textures are well structured. Even edges can be found. The figures 1(a), 1(b), 1(c) and 1(l) give good examples.

2.4 Half-Natural Texture

That leaves the third group of textures, the half-natural textures. These are textures of objects that are natural but formed by man. Examples are a lawn, a corn field, a hedgerow and even a wall made of concrete. If one looks at the

---

[a]The texture types are not to be confused with the texture definitions as described above. Here again it can be observed that the word texture is ill defined and context dependent.

figure 1(e) in detail one will see the structure of wooden planks and pebble stones embedded in the concrete. Another example can be found in figure 1(j).

2.5 Problems with Genuine Texture

Using genuine texture means that a number of problems occur. As the images used are not taken under laboratory conditions they do not have the same scale, intensity and contrast to name only a few parameters. This means that the methods for classifying texture have to be robust in this sense. The aim is to find features that are invariant towards the occurring problems.

3 The System

Figure 2 shows a simplified layout of the Texture Classification System. It is composed of modules and layers. The centerpiece is the Core-System which consists of three modules: the preprocessing methods, the statistical methods and the soft-computing methods. The Core-System classifies the input images and is itself the center module of the Enhanced-System with the image preparation module before and the postprocessing module after it. The Enhanced-System is capable of identifying single texture regions within a larger image. The Optimization System is made up of the genetic algorithm module and the fitness evaluation module. This subsystem can be used for optimization tasks throughout the complete system.

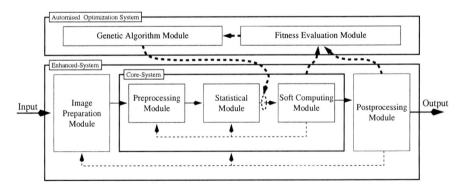

Figure 2. The Texture Classification System.

4   Statistical Feature Extraction

Using statistical methods for feature extraction is one way of classifying texture. Those methods are used in the texture classification system described in this paper.

Preprocessing methods are used to reduce redundant information contained in the texture images. Thus the relevant information can be extracted more easily by using statistical methods.

Currently used methods are a preliminary median filtering followed by a number of image analysis methods. Among these are different kinds of edge detection, gradient extraction, SOBEL filtering, surface and spectral analysis. [15] Next to those standard filter methods the images are processed through wavelets filters [7] and LAWS-measures. [11] The results of these computational steps are not used in the classical sense—it is for example not of interest where edges can be found—but are statistically evaluated.

As the neighbourhood relations of image pixels are of importance high order statistics are used additionally to first order statistical calculations—like mean, variance, skewness, kurtosis. Very good results have been obtained concerning the orientation of similar grey-level pixels within an image. The spatial grey-level dependence (SGLD) matrices used yield potential features, among which are the entropy, correlation, inertia and homogenity. [5]

The combination of all these filters and statistical calculations result in a vast amount of data. But only a fraction of the extracted features provide non-redundant information that is unique to a specific texture. Therefore the number of features has to be reduced to avoid wasting computational resources.

5   Feature Selection using Genetic Algorithms

As the number of features generated in the previous modules of the system is very large—easily exceeding 10^3 or even 10^4—it is necessary to select relevant features for the classification which takes place in the following modules. Doing this manually is not an option as the dimension of the feature plane is by far too large to be visualizable and the possible interconnections between features too complex. Therefore an automatic feature selector has to be included into the system.

Genetic algorithms have the capability of finding very good local or even global optimal solutions in complex data-planes. [14][18] Therefore every feature is associated to one *gene*—a boolean element—and all genes compose the equivalent of a *DNA*. If the gene is set to zero the associated feature is not used in the following modules of the system and it is used if the gene is set to one. One half of the starting population is created randomly, the other half consists of the negated first half. The negation provides an even distribution of zeros and ones for every gene throughout the starting population. In the next step all or some members of the population are used to create a new generation by exchanging parts of the DNA-string. This is called *crossover*. Depending on the way of selection and production of DNAs the population can grow rapidly. Additionally some DNAs can be mutated to avoid getting stuck in a local optimum.

5.1 Single-Cut Crossover

Figure 3 shows graphically how the single-cut crossover works. The spot where the DNA-string is cut is chosen by random. Actually the single-cut crossover is a special two-cut crossover with the second cut always at the end of the DNA-string. The general version of the two-cut crossover is shown in figure 4.

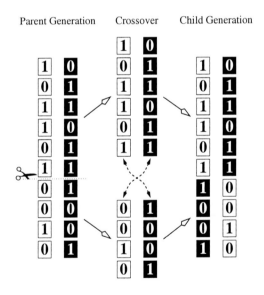

Figure 3. Crossover with single cut.

The two-cut crossover promotes the idea of a ring-DNA—cf. fig. 5—which has no first or last element. The position of all genes are equal.

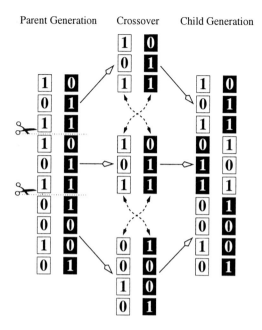

Figure 4. Crossover with two cuts.

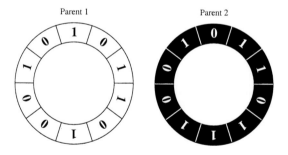

Figure 5. DNA ring.

5.2 Shuffle Crossover

The problem with the formerly mentioned crossover methods is that neighbouring genes will almost always stay together, especially if the DNA-string is very long as in the case of the application described in this paper.

A way of avoiding this is by using the shuffle crossover method. A special shuffle-DNA-string of the same size as the other DNA-strings is created randomly for every new generation. The genes of the parent DNA-strings are exchanged if the according gene of the shuffle-DNA-string is set to one, not exchanged if set to zero. Figure 6 will clarify this procedure.

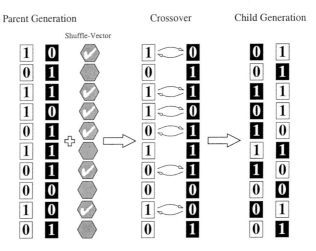

Figure 6. Crossover method with shuffle-DNA-string.

5.3 Mutation and Dimwits

Mutation is needed to avoid finding only local optimal solution. This can happen if throughout the population a certain gene is set to one, or zero accordingly, like the third, sixth or eighth gene in the figure 3. By means of crossover the influence of this gene will never again change, thus only half of the possible solutions can be addressed. Mutation now toggles the influence of a randomly chosen gene from one to zero and vice versa.

Dimwits are DNA-strings with an under par fitness value. Alternatively the least capable may be chosen. One or more dimwits are added to the group of parents and being used for the crossover process. Again the reason is to surpass local optima. A dimwit might has an optimal gene sequence not found in the group of the fittest parents.

Tests have shown that mutation and adding dimwits are important for very long DNA-strings. This is due to the fact that in such cases the population size is for computational reasons usually significantly smaller than the number of genes in a DNA-string.

5.4 Choosing the Parents

A number of different mating procedures can be adopted. The *brute force* method is to mate every individual of the population to all the others. A parent population size of m will produce $m^2 - m$ children, all of which have to be rated for their individual fitness. A way of producing less children—and thus fewer fitness tests—is mating by rank. Possibilities that produce m children are for example

$$\{[1 \infty 2], [3 \infty 4], [5 \infty 6], \cdots, [m - 1 \infty m]\} \tag{1}$$

and

$$\{[1 \infty m], [2 \infty m - 1], [3 \infty m - 2], \cdots, [m/2 \infty m/2 - 1]\} \quad . \tag{2}$$

A variant common in the animal kingdom is to mate the fittest to all others, producing $2(m - 1)$ children:

$$\{[1 \infty 2], [1 \infty 3], [1 \infty 4], \cdots, [1 \infty m]\} \quad . \tag{3}$$

A further variant would be to use the two, three or p fittest individuals for mating with all others:

$$\{[i \infty j]\} \quad \forall \quad i \in \{1, p\}, j \in \{i + 1, m\}, p < m \quad . \tag{4}$$

Here the census will count $p(2m - p - 1)$ children. For $p = m - 1$ this method is identical to the *brute force* method mentioned above.

5.5 Fitness Evaluation

Next to the crossover process itself the fitness evaluation is most important. Fitness evaluation is the performance test of the system using every newly created DNA of the population—the older ones do not have to be tested again—and thus a number of sets of selected features. After those tests only the better DNA-strings—those that yield a better performance of the system which is being optimized—stay in the population and the production of a new population starts again. To keep the population from growing indefinitely only the m fittest individuals are kept. At that point there is no distinction between parents and children.

This process continues as long as the fitness differences between parent and child population are significant for a specified number of generations.

To speed up the fitness testing the new DNA-strings are checked for equal parents or siblings. Tests have shown that even with a very quick fitness test the speed up is significant. Building and testing a complete genealogy-tree will be useful in the case of a longer fitness test. This part has yet to be included into the system.

In the case of this texture classification system the fitness describes the ability to distinguish between different textures. Figure 7 gives an idea how the features that describe a certain texture build a cluster in the feature plane. The aim is to find such a selection of features for which the cluster do not intersect with one another. The better the clusters are kept apart, the easier the classification is.

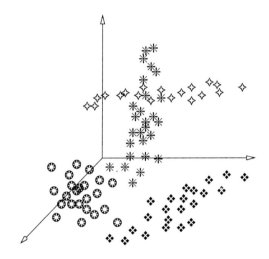

Figure 7. Cluster in a 3D-feature-plane.

6 Classification

As the aim is to find the relevant features to classify the textures a system had to be developed that handles the multi-dimensional feature vectors. Additionally it had to provide the possibility to judge the relevancy of the features. One feasible method is using the cluster analysis for this task. [8] [12] [20]

6.1 Cluster Analysis

The feature vectors—data points in an n dimensional plane—are divided into non-overlapping groups, or clusters, of points. The points within a cluster are "more similar" to one another than to points of other clusters. The term "more similar" means in this context closer by some measure of proximity. This measure can be e. g. the L_p distance:

$$D^p(x_k, x_l) = \left(\sum_{i=1}^{n} |x_{ki} - x_{li}|^p \right)^{\frac{1}{p}} \quad \forall\, p > 0 \quad .$$ (5)

For $p = 1$ this is the Hamming distance, for $p = 2$ the Euclidean distance. Weighing the L_p distance will give the Minkowski distance:

$$D^{\tilde{p}}(x_k, x_l) = \left(\sum_{i=1}^{n} w_i |x_{ki} - x_{li}|^p \right)^{\frac{1}{p}} \quad \forall\, p > 0 \quad .$$ (6)

Every feature vector of a partitioned dataset is assigned to exactly one cluster. Each cluster can be referenced by a single reference point, usually the mean value of all cluster members.

A problem for this kind of sharp clustering is to handle data points that are close to more than one cluster. The figure 8 showing the butterfly-problem gives a graphical example. The central data point (cf. 8(a)) should belong equally to both clusters as shown in 8(c) and not to only one as it is the case when sharp clusters are applied as in figure 8(b). In this example the clusters overlap.

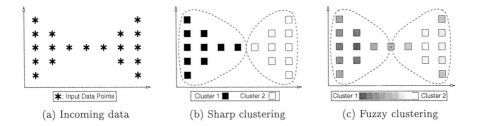

(a) Incoming data   (b) Sharp clustering   (c) Fuzzy clustering

Figure 8. The butterfly-problem.

With increasing numbers of dissimilar textures the chance of clusters overlapping in one or more dimension increases. Therefore new methods had to be adopted to overcome this problem.

6.2 Fuzzy Clustering

Fuzzy logic methods have a potential for handling uncertain knowledge. [16] [22] [24] Thus it is possible to classify texture of which the feature vectors do not point to the center of a certain cluster but into an overlapping area of two or more clusters. [1] [4] [6] [19] Such a texture has a membership value of a certain height for every cluster of the plane. Usually this value equals zero for almost all clusters and obtains a high value for the texture cluster in question. Texture images that have membership values of about equal height have to be treated in a postprocessing system.

One possible fuzzy clustering method is to use the fuzzy c-means algorithm. This is probably the easiest of all fuzzy clustering methods and the base for more specialized versions like the fuzzy c-varieties [2] which uses n dimensional prototypes, the adaptive fuzzy clustering [3] for elliptical cluster shapes and the fuzzy c-spherical shells [10] for hyperspherical shells to name but a few.

Only the fuzzy c-means algorithm shall be explained in some detail in this paper. It is the fuzzy extension of the sharp cluster analysis. As before the distances between all m feature vectors of the training set and the cluster centers v have to be minimized. The difference is that every feature vector gets a membership value μ for every cluster c, noted in the fuzzy partitioning matrix U.

The minimization of the function

$$\min z_w(U, v) = \sum_{k=1}^{m} \sum_{i=1}^{c} \mu_{ik} D_{ik}^p \tag{7}$$

with w being a weighing or fuzzification factor has to obey the supplementary conditions

$$\sum_{i=1}^{c} \mu_{ik} = 1 \quad \forall\, 1 \le k \le m \quad, \tag{8}$$

$$\mu_{ik} \in [0, 1] \quad \forall\, 1 \le i \le c, 1 \le k \le m \quad, \tag{9}$$

$$0 < \sum_{k=1}^{m} \mu_{ik} < m \quad. \tag{10}$$

Finding the optimal fuzzy partition matrix follows the same routine as in the sharp clustering algorithm. After initialization of the number of clusters and the fuzzification factor, the initial cluster centers are determined and the membership values calculated and thus the fuzzy partitioning matrix established. The cluster centers will then be repositioned according to the partitioning matrix and new membership values are calculated. This will continue until the difference between old and new partitioning matrix is small enough.

The problem with this algorithm is of course that the distance measure promotes only certain kinds of compact clusters. Secondly the membership values for feature vectors that are far away from all cluster centers is about equal for all clusters—the membership value function is not monotonous.

Other algorithms that overcome some of these problems (e. g. the algorithm by I. Gath and A. B. Geva [6]) are being included into the system.

6.3 Neural Networks

An alternative to fuzzy clustering is to use neural networks. Widely known backpropagation (BP) networks have been successfully tested for this task. [9] [13] One problem with BP networks is that they are not retrainable, i.e. new classes can not be added without destroying the trained classes. This makes it more difficult and time consuming to expand the number of classes.

A neural network type which overcomes these problems is the adaptive resonance theory (ART) family. [23] Networks of this type can be retrained at any time. These networks are currently included into the system.

A general problem with neural networks is the rather long training time and the great need for computational resources, especially when input (number of features) and output (number of classes) vectors are large in size. In such cases the use of special neural network hardware is almost unavoidable, especially if the network has to be trained again and again to find the optimal feature vector as in the case of this texture classification system. The above mentioned and some other neural network types are being adapted to run on the recently acquired Siemens-Nixdorf Synapse 3•PC neural network hardware.

Once these neural networks are initiated with several clusters of different textures, new texture-images can be identified. Due to the generalization ability of neural networks even textures that are not clearly identifiable get a certain membership degree of several clusters. A post-processing module in the system can handle this information and adjust the pre-processing and statistical modules accordingly.

7 Conclusions

This paper has introduced the use of a complex modular image processing system for texture classification. The necessity and advantages of this approach have been delineated and discussed. Problems associated with the actual textures themselves and other modules of the system have also been addressed.

With an additional border detection algorithm, which is part of the system, it is possible to detect and classify texture areas within a multi-texture image.

This texture classification system can easily be adapted for other tasks, including tasks in the field of medical imaging, remote sensing and quality control.

References

1. J C Bezdek. *Fuzzy Mathematics in Pattern Classification.* PhD Thesis, Cornell University, 1973.

2. J C Bezdek. *Pattern Recognition with Fuzzy Objective Function Algorithms.* Plenum Press, New York, 1981.

3. R N Dave. *Use of the Adaptive Fuzzy Clustering Algorithm to Detect Lines in Digital Images.* Intelligent Robots and Computer Vision VIII, 1192 (2):600–611, 1989.

4. J C Dunn. *A Fuzzy Relative of the ISODATA Process and Its Use in Detecting Compact Well-Separated Clusters.* Journal of Cybernetics, 3/3:32–57, 1973.

5. I M Elfadel, R W Picard. *Gibbs Random Fields, Co-occurrences, and Texture Modeling.* Technical Report # 204, MIT Media Laboratory Perceptual Computing Group, Januar 1993.

6. I Gath, A B Geva. *Unsupervised Optimal Fuzzy Clustering.* IEEE Transactions on Pattern Analysis and Machine Intelligence, 11/7:773–781, 1989.

7. A Graps. *An Introduction to Wavelets.* IEEE Computational Science and Engineering, 2(2), 1995.

8. L Kaufmann, P J Rousseeuw. *Finding Groups in Data: An Introduction to Cluster Analysis.* John Wiley and Sons, New York, 1990.

9. C Klevenhusen. *Texture Analysis with Artificial Neural Networks.* Diplomarbeit, Fachhochschule Braunschweig/Wolfenbüttel / University of Glamorgan, 1996.

10. R Krishnapuram. *Fuzzy Clustering Methods in Computer Vision.* Pro-

ceedings of the 1st European Congress on Intelligent Techniques and Soft Computing, (2):720–730, Aachen, 1993.

11. K I Laws. *Rapid Texture Identification.* SPIE Image Processing for Missile Guidance, 238:376–380, 1980.

12. J MacQueen. *Some Methods for Classification and Analysis of Multivariate Observations.* Proceedings of the 5th Berkeley Symposium, 1:281–297, 1967.

13. S Malon. *Entwicklung eines Systems zur Texturanalyse mittels Wavelet-Transformation und neuronalem Netz für das Bildverarbeitungssystem WiT.* Diplomarbeit, Fachhochschule Braunschweig/Wolfenbüttel, 1997.

14. E Schöneburg, F Heinzmann, S Feddersen. *Genetische Algorithmen und Evolutionsstrategien.* Addison-Wesley, Bonn/Paris/Reading (Mass.), 1994.

15. M Sonka, V Hlavac, R Boyle. *Image Processing, Analysis and Machine Vision.* Chapman & Hall, London, 1993.

16. A Stolpmann. *Fuzzy Logik: Eine Einführung ins Unscharfe.* Diplomarbeit, Fachhochschule Braunschweig/Wolfenbüttel, 1993.

17. A Stolpmann. *Automatic Recognition of Coarse-Grained Non-Regular Structures using Non-Parametric Processing and Soft-Computing Methods – A Texture Classification System.* MPhil/PhD Transfer Document, University of Glamorgan, 1997.

18. A Stolpmann, L S Dooley. *Genetic Algorithms for Automised Feature Selection in a Texture Classification System.* Proceedings of the 4th International Conference on Signal Processing, Beijing, 1998.

19. T Tilli. *Mustererkennung mit Fuzzy-Logik: Analysieren, klassifizieren, erkennen und diagnostizieren.* Franzis-Verlag, München, 1993.

20. R C Tryon. *Cluster Analysis.* Edwards Bros., Ann Arbor, 1939.

21. *Webster's New Encyclopedic Dictionary.* Black Dog & Leventhal Publishers, New York, 1993.

22. L A Zadeh. *Fuzzy Sets.* Information Control, 8:338–353, 1965.

23. A Zell. *Simulation Neuronaler Netze.* Addison-Wesley, Bonn/Paris/Reading (Mass.), 1994.

24. H-J Zimmermann. *Fuzzy Set Theory – And Its Applications.* Kluwer Academic Publishers, Boston/Dordrecht/London, 1991.

AFFINE-INVARIANT TEXTURE CLASSIFICATION USING REGULARITY FEATURES

DMITRY CHETVERIKOV AND ZOLTÁN FÖLDVÁRI

Computer and Automation Research Institute, Budapest, Kende u.13-17, H-1111, Hungary

E-mail: csetverikov@sztaki.hu

Rotation and scale invariant classification has become a well established area of texture analysis. However, content-based image retrieval often requires a higher degree of invariance, since a pattern may appear in a wide range of 3D orientations. This is a new challenge for the existing approaches to texture. It seems that most of them are not prepared to face it. Recently, we have proposed an affine-invariant measure of pattern regularity [7]. In this paper we extend this measure to a feature vector and apply the new approach to invariant classification of regular textures under orthographic projection. 85% accuracy is achieved for 18 patterns.

1 Introduction

Pattern classification is a traditional and fundamental task of texture analysis. The notion of class, that is, which patterns are considered similar and which ones are discriminated, depends on the application problem being solved. In early studies, textures were presented in a normalized orientation, with their anisotropy axes coinciding with the axes of the digital grid. Shift invariance was only required as a natural consequence of the homogeneity underlying the definition of the term 'texture'.

The necessity of a more general invariance was realized in early eighties, when pilot experiments in rotation-invariant texture discrimination were done [6]. However, these attempts attracted limited attention, largely because of the lack of practical demand at that time. Among these initial attempts, the model-based approach [14] should be mentioned.

The spread of multimedia and visual information management lead to a different attitude to the texture classification problem. The task of content-based retrieval in image databases forced the computer vision community to reconsider the original formulation of the problem. Since mid-nineties, several research groups have published their studies in rotation-invariant texture discrimination. A number of novel approaches [17,9,16,25,20,23,5,24] were proposed whose scope and efficiency grew as the work continued. By now, rotation-invariant classification has become a well established area of texture analysis.

Despite this development, it is clear that the task of content-based retrieval requires an even higher degree of invariance. In outdoor imagery the texture being searched often appears in very different views, with weak perspective being a frequent case. The latter is an approximation widely used in vision research, when the size of objects is small compared with the viewing distance. Weak perspective can be interpreted as an orthographic projection onto the image plane followed by an isotropic scaling [18].

When texture classification is to be invariant under weak perspective, the problem should be reconsidered again, since there is a continuum of physically different patterns having the same projection onto the image plane. The situation is exactly the same as with two-dimensional shapes, as discussed by Friedberg [11]. In figure 1, an orthographic projection of a patterns is shown. The nature of projection is readily perceived when the contours of the patterns are shown. When the central part of the projected image is only visible, the single spatial key that remains is the shape of the elements comprising the pattern. When this shape is not specific, the projection is perceived as another homogeneous texture having skewed symmetry.

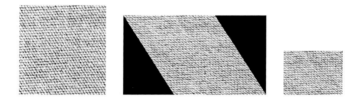

Figure 1. A texture under orthographic projection. Left: texture. Center: an orthographic projection. Right: a subimage of the projection.

In this study, patterns that look the same under weak perspective are not distinguished. Since no additional keys are used, this ambiguity cannot be resolved. The primary application area we aim at is retrieval, where an ambiguity like that usually does not cause a problem, because the goal is to find all potential occurrences of a texture pattern. If it does, additional constraints must be introduced, such as the shape of the textured region.

To our best knowledge, previous work on the problem considered is limited to a few references, such as the early paper [4]. (See also the study [1] where affine invariant segmentation is addressed.) Recently, we proposed a general measure of pattern regularity [7] that is highly invariant and perceptually motivated. In the rest of this paper, we extend this measure to a feature vector, discuss its affine invariance and apply it to texture classification under orthographic projection.

2   Regularity based feature vector

Since the discovery [22] of those fundamental structural features that dominate human texture perception, significant efforts have been put into regularity (periodicity) analysis, with the studies [16,15,13,19] being a few of them. Our approach to affine invariant texture classification exploits the observation that a regular structure is perceived as regular in a wide range of viewing angles. To a certain extent, this is even valid for non-flat structures and changing illumination. A properly defined measure of pattern regularity can therefore serve as a highly invariant, perceptually motivated feature.

The texture descriptor we use stems from the *maximal regularity* feature introduced in our recent paper [7]. The maximal regularity is the maximum value of the *directional regularity* $R(i)$ over all directions i within the pattern. We will first elaborate the computational definition of $R(i)$. This definition differs from the original formulation given in [7]. (The relation between the two formulations is discussed in the appendix.) Based on the directional regularity, we will then introduce the feature vector used in our texture classification experiments.

2.1   The contrast function

Consider a $M \times N$ pixel size digital image $I(m, n)$ and a spacing vector (displacement) (d_x, d_y), where m is the row, n the column, and the conventional co-ordinate system (X, Y) is used. The normalized autocorrelation function of $I(m, n)$ is defined as [21]

$$\rho_{xy}(d_x, d_y) = \frac{1}{S_2} \sum_{m=0}^{M-1} \sum_{n=0}^{N-1} I(m, n) I(m + d_y, n + d_x) \qquad (1)$$

where we denote, for $k = 0, 1, \ldots,$

$$S_k = \sum_{m=0}^{M-1} \sum_{n=0}^{N-1} I^k(m, n) \qquad (2)$$

so that S_0 is the area of the image.

Computing the autocorrelation function by its definition (1) is very time consuming. Fortunately, fast calculation of ρ_{xy} is possible using the well-known relation [21] between the (auto)correlation and the Fourier transform. Applying the fast Fourier transform, FFT, the autocorrelation is readily computed as

$$\rho_{xy}(m, n) = IFFT\left[FFT\left[I(m, n)\right]^* FFT\left[I(m, n)\right]\right], \qquad (3)$$

where $IFFT$ is the inverse FFT.

The FFT can be implemented in different ways. In the implementation we use, the application of (3) yields a matrix whose size is equal to the image size. The latter should be a power of 2. In the rest of this paper, we assume that $N = M = 2^p$, $p = 5, 6, \ldots$. (For $p < 5$, the application of the proposed method is formally possible, but makes no real sense.)

The zero displacement $d_x = d_y = 0$ is in the center of the autocorrelation matrix, which is the origin. The maximum displacement is half the image size, $N/2$. The computation of ρ_{xy} is exemplified in figure 2. The line in figure 2c starts from the origin and indicates the same direction as the one shown in figure 2a.

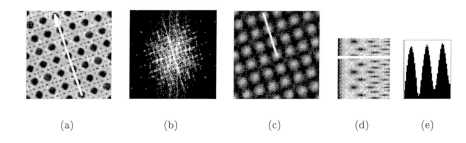

(a)   (b)   (c)   (d)   (e)

Figure 2. Computing the contrast function. (a) A pattern and a direction within this pattern. (b) The DFT of the pattern. (c) The autocorrelation function. (d) The polar interaction map. (e) The contrast function for the direction.

Since we wish to compute pattern regularity for different directions within the pattern, we need a polar representation of the autocorrelation. This representation, $\rho_{pol}(\alpha, d)$, should be defined for arbitrary angle α and magnitude (spacing) d. Given a non-integer location (δ_x, δ_y) in $\rho_{xy}(d_x, d_y)$, $\delta_x = d \cos \alpha$, $\delta_y = -d \sin \alpha$, the value in this location is obtained by the linear interpolation of the four neighboring elements. Note that α and d are continuous, independent parameters, which makes the proposed regularity measure operational.

Using the interpolation, $\rho_{pol}(\alpha, d)$ is computed on the polar grid (α_i, d_j), where $\alpha_i = \Delta\alpha \cdot i$, $d_j = \Delta d \cdot j$. The resulting matrix is denoted by $\rho_{pol}(i, j)$. Normally, we set $\Delta d = 1$ and let the spacing d go up to the maximum possible value $N/2$. It is assumed that $N/2$ covers at least two periods of the pattern. $0 \leq \alpha_i \leq 2\pi$, while the angular resolution $\Delta\alpha$ is task-dependent. In the classification experiments, $\Delta\alpha = 1°$, which provides a sufficient degree of stability under rotation.

The autocorrelation function is normalized: $\rho_{pol}(i,j) \in [0,1]$. By tradition, we use the negated version of the function and call it polar *interaction map* [9,7,8]:

$$M_{pol}(i,j) = 1 - \rho_{pol}(i,j) \qquad (4)$$

In the interaction map, the dark points indicate the periodicity vectors of a structure. An example of a polar map is shown in figure 2d. Relations between the current and the earlier [9,7,8] definitions of the interaction map are discussed in the appendix.

A row of $M_{pol}(i,j)$ is called a *contrast function*. This name reflects the close relation between the autocorrelation and the mean square gray-level difference (contrast), which is elaborated in the appendix. A contrast function $F_i(d)$ shows the variation of contrast with spacing d along a given direction i. An example of a contrast function in displayed in figure 2e. This profile depicts the row marked in figure 2d; the row is, in turn, the cross-section of the (negated) autocorrelation along the line shown in figure 2c.

2.2 Computing the directional regularity

Let us now proceed to the definition of the regularity measure for a direction $i = 1, 2, \ldots, N_\alpha$. ($N_\alpha = 2\pi/\Delta\alpha$ is the number of the directions considered.) The definition is based on the contrast function $F_i(d)$.

To understand the motivations, suppose that one computes the contrast function for the direction of a periodicity vector of the pattern. Figure 3 illustrates results one will typically obtain for patterns with different degrees of regularity. As pointed out by Conners and Harlow [10], a periodic structure will give a contrast function with deep and periodic minima. Our definition of regularity quantifies this property. The definition takes into account that, in general, the shape of the period can be more complex: it may have local minima that indicate the presence of a hierarchical structure.

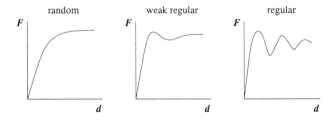

Figure 3. Typical contrast functions of a random, a weak regular and a regular pattern.

For an angle i, the *directional regularity* is defined as

$$R(i) = [R_{int}(i) \cdot R_{pos}(i)]^2, \tag{5}$$

where the $R_{int}(i)$ and $R_{pos}(i)$ are the *intensity regularity* and the *position regularity*, respectively. $R_{pos}(i)$ reflects the regularity (periodicity) of the layout of the elements comprising the pattern, while $R_{int}(i)$ indicates how regular (stable) the intensity of the elements is. The algorithm that computes $R_{int}(i)$ and $R_{pos}(i)$ is described below. For simplicity of notation, we will omit here the direction index i.

Figure 4 illustrates the computation of R for a quasi-periodic contrast function $F(d)$ having a local minimum within the period. When searching for periodicity, two cases are considered. In the normal case (figure 4a) the depths of the global minima decrease monotonically with d. The special case (figure 4b) accounts for possible inhomogeneity of the pattern, when the monotonicity may not hold. The algorithm consists of three procedures and operates as follows.

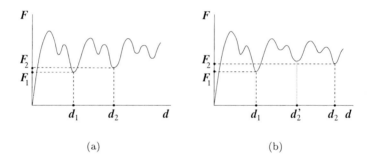

(a) (b)

Figure 4. Computing the regularity measure. (a) Normal case. (b) Special case.

Procedure 1. Finding extrema of $F(d)$.

1. Apply median filter of width 3 to $F(d)$ to remove noisy extrema. Denote the original non-filtered function by $F_0(d)$.

2. Find the extrema of the filtered function $F(d)$, excluding the points $d = 0$ and $d = d_{max}$. (We use the descending component analysis [12].) Denote the numbers of minima and maxima by N_{min} and N_{max}, respectively.

Procedure 2. Computing intensity regularity R_{int}.

1. Compute the (right-side) amplitude of each maximum as follows: starting from a maximum, move right until a higher maximum is found, then store the lowest minimum in this interval; take the difference between the initial maximum and this lowest minimum.

2. Select the maximum (d'_{max}, F'_{max}) having the largest amplitude $F'_{max} - F'_{min}$, where F'_{min} is the lowest minimum assigned to F'_{max}.

3. Rectify F'_{max} by searching $F_0(d)$ for an even higher value in the ± 2 point vicinity of d'_{max}. Set F'_{max} to the highest value found in this vicinity.

4. Rectify F'_{min} is a similar way, but by this time searching for a lower value.

5. Compute the intensity regularity

$$R_{int} = 1 - \frac{F'_{min}}{F'_{max}} \qquad (6)$$

Procedure 3. Computing position regularity R_{pos}.

1. If only one minimum exists ($N_{min} = 1$), find the position d_{max} of the highest maximum and the position $d_1 > d_{max}$ of the lowest minimum after d_{max}, then set

$$R^1_{pos} = 1 - \frac{|d_1 - 2d_{max}|}{d_1} \qquad (7)$$

and stop. Otherwise ($N_{min} > 1$), select the two lowest minima (d_1, F_1) and (d_2, F_2), $d_1 < d_2$, and continue.

2. If there is no minimum between d_1 and d_2 (normal case), compute

$$R_{pos} = 1 - |1 - 2\gamma| \qquad (8)$$

where

$$\gamma = \frac{d_1}{d_2}, \quad 0 < \gamma < 1$$

Otherwise (special case), consider also

$$R'_{pos} = \begin{cases} 1 - |1 - 3\gamma| & \text{if } 1 - |1 - 3\gamma| \geq 0, \\ 0 & \text{otherwise} \end{cases} \qquad (9)$$

and select the larger of R_{pos} and R'_{pos}.

The regularities are normalized so that $R_{int} \in [0,1]$ and $R_{pos} \in [0,1]$. By default, $R_{int} = R_{pos} = 0$ if $N_{min} = 0$ or $N_{max} = 0$.

The median filtering in procedure 1 removes false spike-like extrema, but it also smoothes and shifts the true ones. The correction steps 3 and 4 in procedure 2 restore the original amplitude. A small shift does not affect R_{int} and is currently neglected in R_{pos}.

In procedure 3 (step 2), two alternatives are considered: d_2 is either the second or the third period. (See figures 4a and 4b, respectively.) The corresponding functions (8) and (9) penalize deviations from periodicity. They can be rewritten as

$$R_{pos} = \begin{cases} 2\gamma & \text{if } 0 < \gamma \leq 1/2, \\ 2 - 2\gamma & \text{if } 1/2 < \gamma < 1 \end{cases} \tag{10}$$

$$R'_{pos} = \begin{cases} 3\gamma & \text{if } 0 < \gamma \leq 1/3, \\ 2 - 3\gamma & \text{if } 1/3 < \gamma \leq 2/3, \\ 0 & \text{if } 2/3 < \gamma < 1 \end{cases} \tag{11}$$

R_{pos} and R'_{pos} are piecewise-linear in γ, as depicted in figure 5. R_{pos} penalizes deviations from $d_2 = 2d_1$, R'_{pos} from $d_2 = 3d_1$. To avoid negative values, R'_{pos} is set to 0 when d_2 falls far from $3d_1$ ($d_2 < 1.5d_1$).

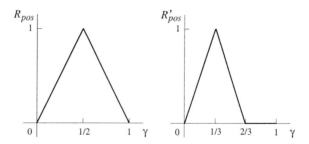

Figure 5. Plots of the functions (10) and (11).

Note that both R_{int} and R_{pos} are invariant to scaling of d. This is important for the affine invariance of regularity.

2.3 Defining the regularity feature vector

The relevant maxima of the directional regularity $R(i)$ indicate those specific, dominant directions within the texture that exhibit stronger periodicity. While the shape of this cyclical function changes under weak perspective, the order of the relevant maxima, their number and height tend to be quite stable, as illustrated in figure 6. This is because pattern regularity in a (physical) dominant direction is preserved: affine transformation preserves both collinearity and periodicity. The largest of the maxima, the maximal regularity, is particularly characteristic and reflects the overall regularity as perceived by a human observer in a view-independent way.

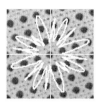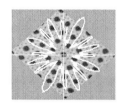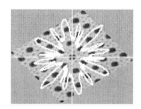

Figure 6. Polar plots of $R(i)$ for three projections of a pattern. The dominant maxima are preserved.

We define a regularity feature vector based on a sequence of the relevant maxima of $R(i)$. The affine invariance of the features stems from the transformation properties of the autocorrelation function, which will be studied in section 3.

Denote by T_k the sequence of the local maxima values of $R(i)$, where $k = 1, 2, \ldots, K$ is the index of the maxima in the sequence. The positions of T_k within $R(i)$ are not retained: their order only matters. To select the relevant maxima, we simply threshold the regularity at a value T_{thr} and discard the low maxima $T_k < T_{thr}$. Previously, it was experienced [7] that $R(i)$ exceeding $R_{thr} = 0.25$ indicates the presence in the pattern of visually perceived periodicity. This ensures that the contrast function is quasi-periodic and fits the model discussed in section 2.2. To cope with weak structures, we allow some room for variation of T_k below R_{thr} and set $T_{thr} = 0.15$.

Denote the thresholded maxima sequence by T'_k, $k = 1, 2, \ldots, K'$. The *feature vector* Φ_l we use consists of 4 components: the largest value M_R, the mean μ_R, the variance σ_R^2, and the density of maxima ν, defined as follows:

$$M_R = \max_k \{T'_k\} \qquad \mu_R = \frac{\sum_k T'_k}{K'} \qquad (12)$$

$$\sigma_R^2 = \frac{\sum_k (\mu_R - T'_k)^2}{K'(K' - 1)} \qquad \nu = \frac{K'}{N_\alpha}. \qquad (13)$$

Since $R(i) \in [0, 1]$, $0 \leq \mu_R \leq M_R \leq 1$, with 0 indicating a random, 1 a highly regular pattern.

3 Affine invariance of regularity

In this section we discuss the affine invariance of the regularity features. For this purpose, let us first investigate the affine transformation of the autocorrelation function. Affine theorem for the continuous two-dimensional Fourier transform has recently been formulated by Bracewell et al in the communication [2]. Here, a similar derivation is applied to the autocorrelation.

Consider a continuous image function $f(x, y)$ that is zero outside a finite domain Q. The (continuous) autocorrelation function $\rho(u, v)$ of $f(x, y)$ is defined by

$$\rho(u, v) = \frac{1}{S_2} \int_{-\infty}^{+\infty} \int_{-\infty}^{+\infty} f(x, y) f(x + u, y + v) \, dx \, dy = \frac{1}{S_2} \varrho(u, v) \qquad (14)$$

where for $k = 0, 1, \ldots$

$$S_k = \int_{-\infty}^{+\infty} \int_{-\infty}^{+\infty} f^k(x, y) \, dx \, dy \qquad (15)$$

and $\varrho(u, v)$ is the unnormalized autocorrelation. (Compare with the discrete version (1).)

The affine co-ordinate transformation is given by

$$x' = ax + by + c \qquad y' = dx + ey + f, \qquad (16)$$

or, in matrix notation:

$$\mathbf{x}' = \mathbf{A}\mathbf{x} + \mathbf{t}, \qquad (17)$$

where

$$\mathbf{x} = \begin{bmatrix} x \\ y \end{bmatrix} \qquad \mathbf{A} = \begin{bmatrix} a & b \\ d & e \end{bmatrix} \qquad \mathbf{t} = \begin{bmatrix} c \\ f \end{bmatrix}$$

It is assumed that $\Delta = \det \mathbf{A} = ae - bd \neq 0$. The unnormalized autocorrelation of the affine transformed image is

$$\varrho'(u, v) = \int_{-\infty}^{+\infty} \int_{-\infty}^{+\infty} f(x', y') f(x' + u', y' + v') \, dx \, dy \qquad (18)$$

Here $\mathbf{u}' = \mathbf{A}\mathbf{u} + \mathbf{t}$. Using the Jacobian relation $dx' \, dy' = |\Delta| \, dx \, dy$ and recalling that $f(x, y)$ is zero outside a finite area, we obtain

$$\varrho'(u, v) = \frac{1}{|\Delta|} \int_{-\infty}^{+\infty} \int_{-\infty}^{+\infty} f(x', y') f(x' + u', y' + v') \, dx' \, dy'$$
$$= \frac{1}{|\Delta|} \varrho(u', v') \qquad (19)$$

From (15) and (19) it follows that $S_2' = S_2/|\Delta|$, hence for the normalized autocorrelation (14) we have

$$\rho'(u,v) = \rho(u',v') \tag{20}$$

In other words, the autocorrelation function transforms as its spacing vector. This simple form of transformation is an advantage of working in the image domain. In the frequency domain the transformation is much more complicated [2].

To better understand the meaning of (20), consider figure 7. In the first row, a pattern is affine-transformed and the autocorrelation of the transformed pattern is computed. In the second row, the autocorrelation of the initial pattern is computed, then affine-transformed. The last picture compares the two results, which are identical up to minor differences originating from the digital nature of the images.

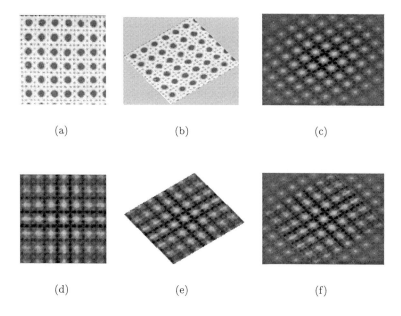

Figure 7. Autocorrelation function under affine transformation. (a) A pattern. (b) An affine transformation of the pattern. (c) The autocorrelation of (b). (d) The autocorrelation of the pattern (a). (e) The affine transformation of (d). (f) Image (e) overlaid on (c).

As discussed by Mundy and Zisserman [18], weak perspective can be viewed as a special case of affine transformation. Weak perspective can be represented as an orthogonal transformation followed by an isotropic scaling, while in an affine transformation the image co-ordinates are scaled differently (anisotropic scaling). However, all the three transformations are linear. In a flat pattern, collinear points remain collinear. Parallelism and periodicity are preserved. Given the relation (20), it is clear that in the continuous case a contrast function undergoes scaling of its argument, a transformation to which the directional regularity measure (5) is invariant, since R_{int} and R_{pos} are so. (See equations (6) and (7–9).)

In digital patterns, the invariance of regularity assigned to a given direction is not strict. In addition, the regularity feature vector is computed for a polar sampling of limited resolution. There is always some variation in the relevant regularity maxima T'_k and the feature values, when they are computed for different views of a pattern. This variation can be observed in figure 6. However, the stability may be sufficient for a number of tasks, including affine invariant classification of textures.

4 Classification experiments

Eighteen structured textures from the album [3] were used in the tests. The patterns selected have $M_R > 0.25$, that is, they possess at least weak regularity. Each initial texture image of 512×512 pixel size was divided into 9 non-overlapping subimages 170×170 size each, and random orthographic projections were computed for 8 of them within the $\pm 40°$ range of the 3 rotation angles. The ninth subimage was left unrotated. No scaling was done because the initial resolution of the test images did not allow for scaling down the images without loss of relevant structural details, especially when a pattern already shrinks due to the orthographic projection. Samples of the 18 classes are displayed in figure 8.

The leave-one-out classification test was carried out based on the nearest class. The test runs as follows. Given a class represented by 9 samples, one of the samples is selected. The other 8 samples are used as the learning samples and the mean values of the four features are computed for these 8 samples. The mean feature values for each of the other 17 classes are computed for all 9 samples. Then the distance between the selected sample s with feature vector $\Phi_l(s)$ and a class c represented by its mean feature vector $\overline{\Phi_l}(c)$ is computed as

$$D(s,c) = \sum_{l=1}^{4} w_l \cdot \left| \Phi_l(s) - \overline{\Phi_l}(c) \right| \qquad (21)$$

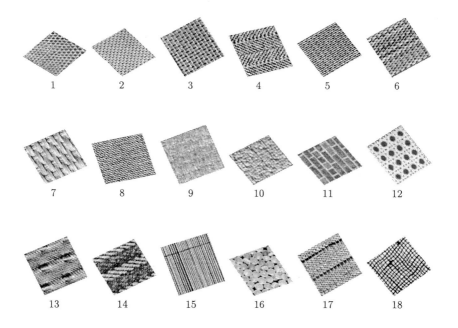

Figure 8. Samples of the test patterns.

where the weights w_l were set empirically as $w_1 = 1$, $w_2 = 2$, $w_3 = 4$, $w_4 = 2$.

The sample s is classified as belonging to the nearest class n: $D(s, n) < D(s, c)$ for all $c \neq n$. This procedure is repeated for each sample of each class. To account for different pattern orientations, the leave-one-out test was performed 200 times, each time with new, randomly generated orientations.

Table 1 is a sample confusion matrix C_{pq} obtained in one of the 200 tests. C_{pq} shows the number of times a sample from class p was classified as belonging to class q, with the off-diagonal elements being misclassifications. (See figure 8 for the order of the classes.) In this particular test, the classification accuracy was 87.65%, which is above the average.

The average accuracy of the 200 tests was 84.82%, the standard deviation 3.18%. The maximum accuracy achieved in an individual test was 89.51%, the minimum 80.86%. The results are reasonable for a pilot attempt, taking into account the high degree of variation due to the spatial rotation.

Table 1. A sample confusion matrix.

true	1	2	3	4	5	6	7	8	9	10	11	12	13	14	15	16	17	18
1	**8**	0	0	0	0	0	1	0	0	0	0	0	0	0	0	0	0	0
2	0	**7**	1	0	0	1	0	0	0	0	0	0	0	0	0	0	0	0
3	0	1	**8**	0	0	0	0	0	0	0	0	0	0	0	0	0	0	0
4	0	0	0	**8**	0	1	0	0	0	0	0	0	0	0	0	0	0	0
5	0	0	0	0	**9**	0	0	0	0	0	0	0	0	0	0	0	0	0
6	0	0	0	0	0	**9**	0	0	0	0	0	0	0	0	0	0	0	0
7	0	0	0	0	0	0	**7**	0	0	0	0	0	1	0	0	0	0	1
8	0	0	1	0	0	0	0	**8**	0	0	0	0	0	0	0	0	0	0
9	0	0	0	0	0	0	0	0	**8**	1	0	0	0	0	0	0	0	0
10	0	0	0	0	0	0	0	0	0	**8**	0	0	1	0	0	0	0	0
11	0	0	0	0	0	0	0	0	0	0	**8**	0	0	0	0	0	0	1
12	0	0	0	0	0	0	0	0	0	0	0	**9**	2	0	0	0	0	0
13	0	0	0	0	0	0	0	0	0	0	1	0	**8**	0	0	0	0	0
14	0	0	0	0	0	0	0	0	0	0	0	0	0	**8**	0	0	1	0
15	0	0	0	0	0	0	0	0	0	0	0	1	0	0	**8**	0	0	0
16	0	0	0	0	0	0	0	0	0	0	1	0	0	0	0	**8**	0	0
17	0	0	0	0	0	0	0	0	0	0	0	0	0	0	3	0	0	**6**	0
18	1	0	0	0	0	0	1	0	0	0	0	0	0	0	0	0	0	**7**

5 Discussion and outlook

Additional experiments were carried out to better understand the potential and the limits of the proposed approach. Different combinations of the four regularity features (12),(13) were tested and the classification results compared. The results indicate that, despite the obvious correlation between the features, the overall accuracy is the best when all the four features are used.

At the same time, the classification procedure is a subject of further research. Figure 9 shows two additional regular textures. Their inclusion in the test dataset decreases the accuracy of the sample test (table 1) from 87.65% to 82.78%, as both patterns are misclassified 5 of 9 times. Further extension of the dataset would probably lead to further decrease of accuracy. The message is that regularity alone is not sufficient for reliable discrimination of a large number of textures.

Another limitation of regularity is that two different images of the same physical structure will be discriminated if one of the images is considerably

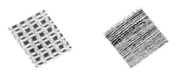

Figure 9. Two additional textures.

deteriorated by noise, blur and other distortions, while the other is not. Obviously, the two images will have different regularities. This is exemplified by the patterns 2 and 3 of the classification test. (See figure 8 and table 1.) The two images show the same woven aluminum wire, but photographed and digitized under different conditions. The patterns are visually different and are classified as such. Note that this classification result is not due to the different shadowing, which has limited effect on the regularity of the almost flat wire structure.

Since we intend to use the proposed approach in an image retrieval system, the estimated probability of the true class to be among the K nearest classes was calculated. That is, for each sample s the distances $D(s, s'), s \neq s'$ defined as

$$D(s, s') = \sum_{l=1}^{4} w_l \cdot \left| \Phi_l(s) - \Phi_l(s') \right| \tag{22}$$

were ranked and the samples s' giving the K lowest values selected. The weights were the same as in the classification test (21), but this time no learning (calculation of $\overline{\Phi_l}(c)$) was done. For the 18 textures shown in figure 8 this probability was 87.04% for $K = 1$ and 95.06% for $K = 3$. When the two patterns shown in figure 9 are added, these values decrease to 81.11% and 92.22%, respectively. Clearly, much larger database is needed here to obtain statistically significant results.

Online demonstrations of the invariant classification and retrieval are available on the Internet at the web site of the Image and Pattern Analysis (IPAN) Research Group: http://visual.ipan.sztaki.hu.

An open problem is that of selecting the image resolution and the angular resolution parameter $\Delta\alpha$. Weak perspective involves both orthographic projection and scaling. In our tests, scaling was not included since important structural features of fine patterns would be lost at a lower resolution. Regularity is resolution-dependent, which may result in more misclassifications if not taken into account properly.

To roughly estimate the lower limit for resolution, one may consider that the pattern period should be greater than 10 pixels. The width of periodic structural features, for instance, parallel lines, should be at least 2–3 pixels. To make the proposed method more flexible and robust, it is planned to apply a multiscale approach trying to handle the variation of structure with scale.

Acknowledgments

This work is partially supported by the Hungarian Scientific Research Fund under the grant OTKA T026592.

Appendix. Autocorrelation function and moments of GLDH.

In this appendix we discuss the relation between the autocorrelation function and the moments of the gray-level difference histogram GLDH. GLDH is a standard tool of texture analysis [12]. Its entries are the estimated occurrence probabilities of absolute gray-level differences between pixels separated by a given spacing vector. The first and the second moment of GLDH are frequently used as efficient texture features. Our previous definitions of contrast function and regularity [7] were also based on the moments of GLDH. It is instructive to clarify the similarity and the difference between the autocorrelation and the moments, that is, between the alternative definitions of regularity.

In the continuous case, the autocorrelation function is defined by equation (14). Similarly, consider again a continuous image $f(x,y)$ which is zero outside a finite domain Q. The k-th order moment of GLDH is expressed as

$$
\begin{aligned}
M_k(u,v) &= \frac{1}{S_0} \int_{-\infty}^{+\infty} \int_{-\infty}^{+\infty} |f(x,y) - f(x+u, y+v)|^k \, dx \, dy \\
&= \frac{1}{S_0} m_k(u,v)
\end{aligned}
\tag{23}
$$

where $m_k(u,v)$ is the unnormalized moment and S_k are defined by (15); in particular, S_0 is the area of Q.

The moments describe the gray-level difference, or 'contrast', as a function of spacing. The name 'contrast feature' has been traditionally used for $M_1(u,v)$ or $M_2(u,v)$ computed for small spacings $u, v = \pm 1$. Calculating $M_2(u,0)$ in a larger interval of spacings, Conners and Harlow [10] observed the quasi-periodicity of contrast the function discussed in section 2.1.

In simplified notation, the unnormalized second moment can be rewritten as

$$m_2(u,v) = \int \int f^2(x,y)\, dx\, dy + \int \int f^2(x+u, y+v)\, dx\, dy$$
$$- 2 \int \int f(x,y) f(x+u, y+v)\, dx\, dy$$

Since $f(x,y)$ is zero outside a finite area, the first two integrals are equal and

$$m_2(u,v) = 2 \int \int f^2(x,y)\, dx\, dy - 2 \int \int f(x,y) f(x+u, y+v)\, dx\, dy \tag{24}$$
$$= 2\big[S_2 - \varrho(u,v)\big],$$

where $\varrho(u,v)$ is the unnormalized autocorrelation (14). For the normalized moment, we obtain

$$M_2(u,v) = \frac{2}{S_0}\big[S_2 - \varrho(u,v)\big] = \frac{2S_2}{S_0}\Big[1 - \frac{\varrho(u,v)}{S_2}\Big] = \frac{2S_2}{S_0}\big[1 - \rho(u,v)\big]$$
$$= \frac{2S_2}{S_0} M_{xy}(u,v) \tag{25}$$

That is, the second moment $M_2(u,v)$ is equal, up to a constant factor, to the autocorrelation-based interaction map $M_{xy}(u,v) = 1 - \rho(u,v)$.

In practice, the integration in (23) is substituted by summation in a finite digital image. When $f(x,y)$ is a homogeneous texture and the maximum spacing considered is much smaller than the size of Q, the relation (25) is valid as an approximation.

The spatial structures of $M_1(u,v)$, $M_2(u,v)$ and $M_{xy}(u,v)$ are similar, as illustrated in figure 10. Any of them can be used for regularity analysis. The advantage of $M_{xy}(u,v)$ is its fast, *FFT* based implementation. The moments are much more precise at small spacings, which is important for random patterns. Moreover, due to its additivity, $M_1(u,v)$ can be implemented in a sliding window as a running filter [8].

References

1. C. Ballester and M. Gonzalez. Affine Invariant Texture Segmentation and Shape From Texture by Variational Methods. *Journal of Mathematical Imaging and Vision*, 9:141–171, 1998.
2. R.N. Bracewell, K.-Y. Chang, A.K. Jha and Y.-H. Wang. Affine Theorem for Two-Dimensional Fourier Transform. *Electronics Letters*, 29:304, 1993.

86

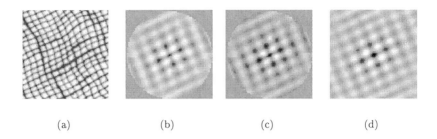

(a)   (b)   (c)   (d)

Figure 10. (a) A pattern. (b) $M_1(u,v)$. (c) $M_2(u,v)$. (d) $M_{xy}(u,v)$.

3. P. Brodatz. *Textures: a Photographic Album for Artists and Designers.* Dover, New York, 1966.
4. S. Chang, L.S. Davis, S.M. Dunn, J.O. Eklundh, and A. Rosenfeld. Texture Discrimination by Projective Invariants. *Pattern Recognition Letters*, 5:337–342, 1987.
5. J.L. Chen and A. Kundu. Rotation and Gray Scale Transform Invariant Texture Identification Using Wavelet Decomposition and Hidden Markov Model. *IEEE Trans. on Pattern Analysis and Machine Intelligence*, 16:208–214, 1998.
6. D. Chetverikov. Experiments in the Rotation-Invariant Texture Discrimination Using Anisotropy Features. In *Proc. International Conf. on Pattern Recognition*, pages 1071–1073, 1982.
7. D. Chetverikov. Pattern Regularity as a Visual Key. In *Proc. British Machine Vision Conf.*, pages 23–32, 1998.
8. D. Chetverikov. Texture Analysis Using Feature Based Pairwise Interaction Maps. *Pattern Recognition*, 32:487–502, 1999.
9. D. Chetverikov and R.M. Haralick. Texture Anisotropy, Symmetry, Regularity: Recovering Structure from Interaction Maps. In *Proc. British Machine Vision Conf.*, pages 57–66, 1995.
10. R.W. Conners and C.A. Harlow. Toward a Structural Textural Analyzer Based on Statistical Methods. *Computer Graphics and Image Processing*, 12:224–256, 1980.
11. S.A. Friedberg. Finding Axis of Skewed Symmetry. *Computer Vision, Graphics and Image Processing*, 34:138–155, 1986.
12. R. M. Haralick and L. G. Shapiro. *Computer and Robot Vision*, volumes I-II. Addison-Wesley, 1992-1993.
13. H.-B.Kim and R.-H. Park. Extracting Spatial Arrangement of Structural

Textures Using Projection Information. *Pattern Recognition*, 25:237–245, 1992.

14. R.L. Kashyap and A. Khotanzad. A Model-Based Method for Rotation Invariant Texture Classification. *IEEE Trans. on Pattern Analysis and Machine Intelligence*, 8:472–481, 1986.

15. H.C. Lin, L.L. Wang, and S.N. Yang. Extracting Periodicity of a Regular Texture Based on Autocorrelation Functions. *Pattern Recognition Letters*, 18:433–443, 1997.

16. F. Liu and R.W. Picard. Periodicity, Directionality, and Randomness: Wold Features for Image Modeling and Retrieval. *IEEE Trans. Pattern Analysis and Machine Intelligence*, 18:722–733, 1996.

17. S.V.R. Madiraju and C.C. Liu. Rotation Invariant Texture Classification Using Covariance. In *First IEEE International Conference on Image Processing*, volume II, pages 655–659, 1994.

18. J.L. Mundy and A. Zisserman. Projective Geometry in Machine Vision. In J.L. Mundy and A. Zisserman, editors, *Geometric Invariance in Computer Vision*, pages 463–534. MIT Press, 1992.

19. J. Parkkinen, K. Selkainaho, and E. Oja. Detecting Texture Periodicity From the Cooccurrence Matrix. *Pattern Recognition Letters*, 11:43–50, 1990.

20. M. Pietikäinen, T. Ojala and Z. Xu. Rotation-Invariant Texture Classification Using Feature Distributions. *Pattern Recognition*, 33:43–52, 2000.

21. I. Pitas. *Digital Image Processing Algorithms*. Prentice Hall, 1993.

22. A.R. Rao and G.L. Lohse. Identifying High Level Features of Texture Perception. *CVGIP: Image Processing*, 55:218–233, 1993.

23. T.N. Tan. Rotation Invariant Texture Features and Their Use In Automatic Script Identification. *IEEE Trans. on Pattern Analysis and Machine Intelligence*, 20:751–756, 1998.

24. L.Z. Wang and G. Healey. Using Zernike Moments for the Illumination and Geometry Invariant Classification of Multispectral Texture. *IEEE Transactions on Image Processing*, 7:196–203, 1998.

25. W.R. Wu and S.C. Wei. Rotation and Gray-Scale Transform-Invariant Texture Classification Using Spiral Resampling, Subband Decomposition, and Hidden Markov Model. *IEEE Transactions on Image Processing*, 5:1423–1434, 1996.

ROBUSTNESS OF LOCAL BINARY PATTERN (LBP) OPERATORS TO TILT-COMPENSATED TEXTURES

MARICOR SORIANO, TIMO OJALA AND MATTI PIETIKÄINEN

Machine Vision and Media Processing Unit
Infotech Oulu and Department of Electrical Engineering
P.O. Box 4500 FIN-90014 University of Oulu FINLAND
E-mail: {msoriano,skidi,mkp}@ee.oulu.fi

Texture classifiers are usually trained with samples in some standard position, e.g. surface normal parallel to the camera axis, light source at fixed position. However, the same textures sampled under different conditions are prone to being misclassified because of appearance change. We consider texture images whose surface normals have been tilted $11.25°$ with respect to the camera axis. Local Binary Operators (LBP) are known to perform very well for texture analysis. In this paper we show that LBP outperforms existing texture classifiers when applied to tilted textures and when standard-position textures are used for training. Neglecting self-shadowing and masking effects by considering only small tilt, we show that recovering a frontal view of the texture by stretching the image about the axis of rotation and by transforming the histogram towards the frontal view histogram further improves LBP performance over uncorrected images.

1 Introduction

The appearance of rough textures is strongly influenced by illumination and viewing geometry because of the 3-D structure of facets making up the surface. The same texture sampled under different illumination or viewing geometry can appear differently. Thus, in general, most texture analysis techniques can only be used if the sample, illumination and viewing conditions are kept constant during training and testing. Research on analysing the appearance of 3-D textures has been performed [3,5,9] and recovering the surface shape from texture is a popular problem [1,7,8]. However, only few papers have been written on geometry invariance in texture classification [2,6].

In the method introduced by Chantler and McGunningle[2], the sample is fixed but the illuminant is rotated about the camera axis causing different shadow patterns. Their solution is to estimate a surface model, generate artificial instances of the texture under different illumination tilts and train the classifier with the simulated data. Their classification results are in close agreement with a classifier trained for each illuminant tilt angle.

Kondepudy and Healey[6] examined color textures and used correlation within and between color bands. Moment invariants derived from these correlations are used as features for classification, and surface orientation parameters can be estimated as well.

We study the case when the illuminant and camera positions are fixed but the sample normal is tilted with respect to the camera axis. Henceforth 'tilt' will mean the angle between the sample normal and the camera axis. For simplicity, we consider small tilt angles and textures with small surface roughness. We assume that surface tilt, camera and illuminant location are known or can be derived by other techniques. These constraints are valid e.g. in many surface inspection applications. Under these conditions, texture images undergo slight geometric distortion and significant brightness change. The performance of a classifier trained with textures in a standard position will then likely degrade when shown tilted versions of the same textures.

An obvious remedy is to recover a frontal view of the tilted texture as a preprocessing step. To test this solution, we developed a simple procedure to transform tilted textures towards the standard position to see if the performance of trained classifiers will improve. The procedure involves geometric correction to account for perpective distortion and histogram transformation to correct for image brightness. Unlike in Chantler and McGunningle's method no retraining of the classifiers was carried out, nor were invariant features derived as in Kondepudy and Healey's method.

Recently, our group developed a nonparametric approach to texture analysis based on simple spatial operators like local binary patterns (LBP) and signed gray level differences. Excellent performance has been shown in various texture classification and segmentation problems [10,11, 12, 13]. We tested our approach using tilted textures and compared results with existing texture analysis techniques. The classifiers were trained using only textures in a standard position. The results indicate how robust a texture analyser is with respect to (slight) changes in imaging geometry, an important attribute in real world applications.

In this paper, we show that, for the small tilt angle case, LBP is most robust in classifying uncorrected tilted textures over existing texture analyzers. A simple image correction improves its classification rate far better than in other texture analyzers.

2 Method

2.1 Local Binary Patterns

Ojala et al. [10] introduced the Local Binary Pattern (LBP) texture operator shown in 1. The original 3x3 neighbourhood is thresholded by the value of the center pixel. The values of the pixels in the thresholded neighbourhood

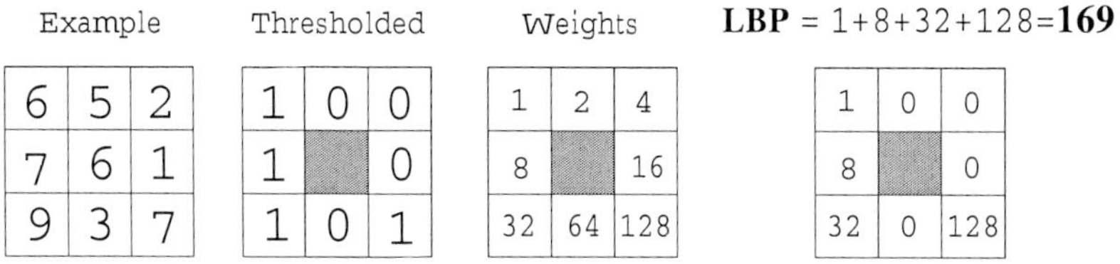

| Example | Thresholded | Weights | **LBP** $= 1+8+32+128=\textbf{169}$ |

6	5	2
7	6	1
9	3	7

1	0	0
1		0
1	0	1

1	2	4
8		16
32	64	128

1	0	0
8		0
32	0	128

Figure 1. Computation of Local Binary Pattern (LBP)

are multiplied by the weights given to the corresponding pixels. Finally, the values of the eight weighted pixels are summed to obtain a number for this neighbourhood. The LBP histogram computed over a region is used as texture description. Because of the LBP design, it is invariant under any monotonic gray scale transformation and provides information about the spatial structure of the local image texture. This is desirable because the average gray level of tilted textures is highly variable. Due to its 3x3 window operation, however, feature distributions may be sensitive to geometric distortion.

2.2   Correction

When non-occluding textures are considered and when the surface normal is tilted from the camera axis by a small angle, we can ignore self-shadowing and masking effects and correct only for foreshortening. Consider patterns spaced D apart in a texture plane with the surface normal **n'** as shown in Figure 2. Let **V** be the camera axis and T the angle between **n'** and **V**. The projected patterns are then spaced by D_f

$$D_f = D\mathbf{n}' \cdot \mathbf{V} = D\cos T. \tag{1}$$

If we have a foreshortened image, we may then transform it back to frontal position by stretching the image by a factor of $1/\cos T$ about its axis of rotation. Nearest neighbour interpolation is then used to assign values in intermediate pixels. Note that this is valid only for small tilt angles. Shadowing and masking effects will dominate for larger tilt angles. It is not advisable to use block bilinear or block bicubic interpolation if the stretching is only along one axis.

When the surface tilts, it tends to look darker if it tilts away from the source or brighter towards the source. To recover the original brightness, the

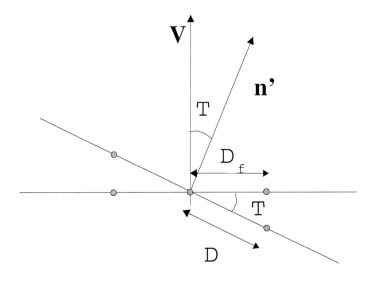

Figure 2. Foreshortening of patterns as seen by camera.

graylevel histogram of the tilted texture is transformed such that its cumulative histogram is equal to the cumulative histogram of the standard position case. This assumes that the histogram of the standard case is known. Van Ginneken and Koenderink [15] have shown that it is possible to determine this histogram, given the current illumination and viewing geometry and the histogram of the present case. To avoid errors that may arise from estimating the standard case histogram we assume that this is exactly known instead of implementing the procedure. Therefore we use the actual histogram of the standard case for brightness correction.

2.3 CURET Database

Figure 3 shows 16 textures from the Columbia - Utrecht (CURET) Database[4] considered for classification. They are polyester (sample 02), leather (sample 05), sandpaper (sample 06), rough paper (sample 12), roof shingle (sample 14), cork (sample 16), rug_a (sample 18), rug_b (sample 19), styrofoam (sample 20), quarry tile (sample 25), loofah (sample 26), slate_a (sample 33), slate_b (sample 34), brick_a (sample 37), brick_b (sample 41) and concrete (sample 49). (Although the correction procedure was intended for non-occluding textures, some of these textures have large height variations.) The CURET Database is unique because each texture has been imaged at 205 different camera and illuminant positions thus capturing the variety of appearances a single texture can take. We chose instances of each texture within which the camera and illuminant were spaced 67.5^o apart ($\theta_v = 0, \theta_i = 67.5^o, \phi_i + \phi_v = 180^o$) with the texture sample normal parallel to camera axis (standard position) and tilted from the camera axis by 11.25^o in the plane of camera and illuminant as shown in Figure 4.

2.4   Classification

LBP histograms for each class were computed from whole images in the standard position. For classification, test images were divided into 64x64 non-overlapping samples. A test sample S was assigned to the class of model M that maximized the log-likelihood measure

$$L(S, M) = \sum_{n=1}^{N} S_n \log M_n \qquad (2)$$

where S_n and M_n are the sample and model probabilities of bin n, respectively.

2.5   Comparative Methods

In addition to LBP, five well-known texture measures were also tested. They are Gaussian Markov Random Fields (GMRF); Gabor filters (GABOR) for 2,4 and 8 pixels and averaged for angles 0, 45, 90 and 135 degrees; fractal dimensions (FRACTAL) computed from 10x10 grids; gray level cooccurence matrices (GLCM) using the Conners-Trivedi-Harlow feature set; and signed gray level differences (DIFFXY) along the horizontal and vertical directions[13]. The first four techniques were implemented using source codes from the publicly available MeasTex website [14] and a multivariate Gaussian classifier was used for classification. For DIFFXY, since it outputs a histogram, Equation 2 was used for classification. Different mask sizes were tried for GMRF (1st to 6th order standard symmetric, and 5 pixel cross-symmetric) and GABOR (from 3x3 up to 17x17 masks). DIFFXY was tested with 8 up to 256 gray levels. It was found that a 3rd order standard symmetric mask for GMRF, a 5x5 mask for GABOR, and 16 graylevels for DIFFXY gave the best overall performance for both standard and tilted images.

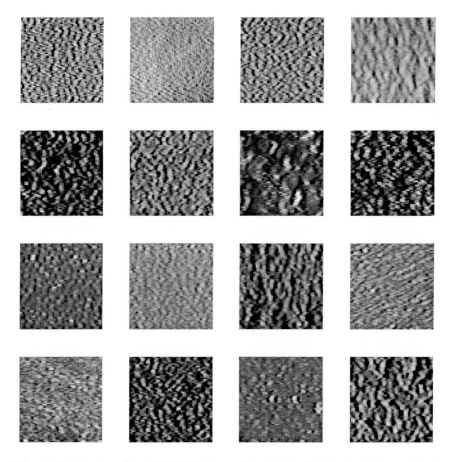

Figure 3. Test textures from CURET database. From left to right, top to bottom, polyester (sample 02), leather (sample 05), sandpaper (sample 06), rough paper (sample 12), roof shingle (sample 14), cork (sample 16), rug_a (sample 18), rug_b (sample 19), styrofoam (sample 20), quarry tile (sample 25), loofah (sample 26), slate_a (sample 33), slate_b (sample 34), brick_a (sample 37), brick_b (sample 41) and concrete (sample 49).

3 Results

Figure 5 shows 64x64 images of sample 06 (sandpaper) in the standard position, tilted by 11.25, frontalized only, and frontalized with histogram correction as discussed in Section 2.2, below each image is its corresponding his-

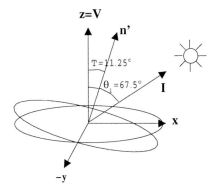

Figure 4. Sampling geometry for standard and tilted texture cases.

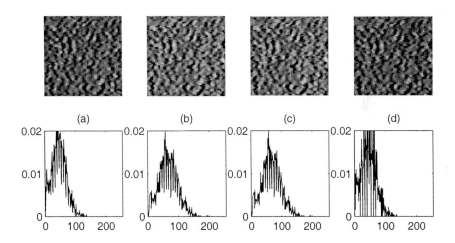

Figure 5. From left to right column:Sample 06 (sandpaper) image and histogram in (a) standard position, (b) tilted, (c) tilt-compensated, (d) tilt-compensated and histogram corrected.

togram. The tilt, in this case, is towards the light source thus the histogram shape shifts towards higher graylevels.

The second column in Table 1 indicates the error rates for each classifier when the the texture analyzer trains on the whole image and is applied to 64x64 cut-outs from the same image. GABOR gives the best recognition (perfect) followed by LBP. The third column shows the error rates when the trained classifier is used on tilted versions of the same texture. Error rates rise drastically for all except LBP. The fourth column shows error rates for geometrically corrected tilted images. Again, LBP improved whereas mixed results are seen from the rest. Despite some decrease in FRACTAL, GLCM and DIFFXY, the error rates are still too high.

There was dramatic improvement in the error rates by just applying histogram correction on the tilted image, as shown in the fifth column. GABOR is found to have the lowest, followed by LBP. Columns 3 to 5 demonstrate that the 5 other texture analysers are sensitive to gray level variations. LBP has an advantage over the 5 other texture analysers for being invariant to grayscale transformations because significant improvement in classification is achieved by a simple geometric correction.

Finally, tilt-compensation and histogram correction are combined and error rates for such treated textures are shown in column 6. The best performance is from GABOR followed by LBP.

While GABOR shows a smaller error rate than LBP after histogram correction is applied, LBP is shown to consistently have only small error in all conditions, particularly for the uncorrected case. In a real world application, if, for example, a texture surface under inspection is slightly tilted, a GABOR-based classifier is more likely to fail than an LBP-based classifier.

We now investigate in more detail the classification results of LBP. Table 2 shows per sample error rates in the same order of columns as in Table 1. Note that most textures are still recognized after tilting. The best case is when geometric correction is followed by histogram correction. Note however that histogram correction alone has almost similar results to the tilted case. This again shows that LBP is invariant to grayscale transformations. This is also proven by the fact that frontalized and front.+hist has almost the same results. Finally, samples 26 and 34 have consistently high error rates even with the standard case. A look at their confusion matrices reveals that sample 26 (loofah) is often mistaken as sample 16 (cork) while sample 34 (slate_b) is often mistaken for sample 41 (brick_b). This implies that these textures have very similar microstructures and represent classes which are difficult for LBP to distinguish. With all the rest of the samples, however, LBP shows excellent recovery.

4 Conclusions

LBP and five other texture measures were tested on tilted and tilt-compensated textures using standard-position textures as training set. LBP

Table 1. Summary of percentage error rates on standard, tilted and compensated textures using different texture analysers

classifier	standard	tilted 11.25°	frontalized	hist only	front.+hist
DIFFXY	5.1	27.8	25.6	12.4	11.4
FRACTAL	15.4	53.2	50.5	19.1	21.8
GABOR	0.0	68.7	70.4	3.2	2.0
GLCM	1.1	62.1	57.7	30.5	37.8
GMRF	1.1	43.5	49.8	11.1	21.8
LPB	0.9	11.7	5.6	8.4	4.3

Table 2. Summary of LBP error rates per sample

sample	standard	tilted 11.25°	frontalized	hist only	front.+hist
02	0.0	100.0	33.3	100.0	31.0
05	0.0	0.0	0.0	0.0	0.0
06	0.0	0.0	0.0	0.0	0.0
12	0.0	0.0	0.0	0.0	0.0
14	0.0	5.7	0.0	0.0	0.0
16	0.0	0.0	0.0	0.0	0.0
18	0.0	0.0	0.0	0.0	0.0
19	0.0	13.3	0.0	13.3	0.0
20	0.0	0.0	0.0	0.0	0.0
25	0.0	2.9	0.0	0.0	0.0
26	10.0	6.7	22.9	6.7	22.9
33	0.0	0.0	0.0	0.0	0.0
34	2.9	23.3	25.7	13.3	11.4
37	0.0	2.9	0.0	0.0	0.0
41	0.0	32.1	5.7	0.0	0.0
49	3.7	14.8	3.7	11.1	3.7

is shown to be the most robust for tilted textures. For small tilt angles T and for textures with small height variations, image distortion due to foreshortening can be compensated for by stretching the image by a factor of $1/\cos T$ about the axis of tilt and using nearest neighbour interpolation to account for the intermediate pixels. Image brightness can be adjusted by transforming graylevels such that the cumulative histogram of the tilted image is equal to the cumulative histogram of the standard position image. An overall improvement in LBP and GABOR classification performance is observed for $T = 11.25^o$ when corrected images are used. Even though GABOR posted smaller error rates than LBP when classifying images with histogram correction, this shows that GABOR is highly sensitive to image brightness variation.

Note that this approach is valid only for small tilts. For larger tilts, appearance change due shadowing and masking will dominate over foreshortening. To extend the image correction to small, arbitrary illumination and viewing angles, the inverse of their affine transformations may be used to even correct for scaling under perspective transformation.

If a simple, physically plausible image correction scheme improves the classification performance of LBP then this suggests that LBP and LBP-like operators can be made robust to texture distortions due to changes in the texture plane.

Our results also indicate that due to shifting grayscale of tilted surfaces, grayscale invariant features like LBP should be preferred over grayscale variant features.

The approach that we took here was to recover a frontal view of the surface so that it can be used with an LBP classifier trained with the standard case. A future goal is also to develop LBP-like operators that can deliver features which are already invariant to surface shape and gray scale transformations.

Acknowledgments

This research received financial support from Infotech Oulu and the Academy of Finland. M. Soriano's permanent address is at the National Institute of Physics, University of the Philippines, Diliman Quezon City, Philippines. Thanks are due to the creators of MeasTex and the CURET Database.

References

1. D. Blostein and N. Ahuja, 'Shape from texture: integrating texture-element extraction and surface estimation', *IEEE Transactions on Pattern Analysis and Machine Intelligence*, **11** 1233-1251 (1989).
2. M.J. Chantler and G. McGunnigle, 'Compensation of illuminant tilt variation for texture classification', *Proc. Image Processing and Its Applications* , 767-771 (1995).
3. K. Dana and S. Nayar, 'Histogram model for 3-D textures' *Proc. Computer Vision and Pattern Recognition (CVPR)*, 618-624 (1998).

4. K. Dana, S. Nayar, B. van Ginneken and J. Koenderink, 'Reflectance and texture of real-world surfaces', *Proc. CVPR*, 151-157 (1997).
5. J.J. Koenderink and A.J. van Doorn, 'Illuminance textre due to surface mesostructure', *J. Optical Society of America A(JOSA A)*, **13** 452-463 1996.
6. R. Kondepudy and G. Healey, 'Use of invariants for recognition of three-dimensional color textures', *JOSAA*, **11** 3037-3049 (1994).
7. J. Krumm and S. Shafer, 'Shape from periodic texture using the spectrogram', *CVPR*, 284-301 (1992).
8. J. Malik and R. Rosenholtz, 'A differential method for computing local shape-from-texture for planar and curved surfaces', *CVPR*, 267-273 (1993).
9. S. Nayar and M. Oren, 'Visual appearance of matte surfaces', *Science*, **267** 1153-1156 1995.
10. T. Ojala, M. Pietikäinen and D. Harwood, 'A comparative study of texture measures with classification based on feature distributions', *Pattern Recognition*, **29** 51-59 (1996).
11. T. Ojala, M. Pietikäinen and J. Nisula, 'Determining composition of grain mixtures by texture classification based on feature distributions', *Intl. J. Pattern Recognition Artif. Intell.*, **10** 73-82 (1996).
12. T.Ojala and M. Pietikäinen, 'Unsupervised texture segmentation using feature distributions', *Pattern Recognition*, **32** 477-486 (1999).
13. T. Ojala, K.Valkealahti, E. Oja and M. Pietikäinen. 'Texture discrimination with multidimensional distributions of signed gray level differences', Submitted for review 1999.
14. G. Smith and I. Burns, 'Measuring texture classification algorithms', *Pattern Recognition Letters* , **18** 1495-1501 (1997).
15. B. Van Ginneken and J. Koenderink, 'Texture histograms as a function of irradiation and viewing direction', *Intl. J. Computer Vision*, **31** 169-184 (1999).

AN INVESTIGATION INTO COLOUR TEXTURE SIMILARITY

G. D. FINLAYSON AND G.Y. TIAN
School of Information Systems, University of East Anglia, Norich, NR4 7TJ, UK
E-mails: {graham, g.y.tian}@sys.uea.ac.uk

Colour and texture are basic features used in many visual processing applications, including machine vision, image retrieval and scene analysis. However, for the most part they have been examined in isolation. We are investigating how this gap might best be filled. In this paper, we report on psychophysical experiments that we carried out to investigate how human observers judge colour texture. Observers were presented with pairs of colourful textures and rated their similarity by scoring a number from 1 to 100. The set of all paired comparisons for a data set of 32 textures led to complete set of similarity judgements and these were placed in a distance matrix. Distance matrices for different observers were then analysed using the technique of MDS (Multi-dimensional scaling). MDS attempts to interpret the similarity distance as the Euclidean distance of points in colour-texture space. That is, MDS returns one point per texture with the Euclidean distance between points correlating with the similarities in the distance matrix.

Our initial pilot experiments appear to show a large variance in the types of colour texture features that observers use for judging similarity. For some observers, the colour aspect of textures is very important yet other observers match almost entirely on pattern. Our experiments appear to indicate that colour texture, interpreted in the context of our own visual system, is either observer or task dependent. We discuss the implications of this for computer vision applications.

1 Introduction

Texture is an important cue in visual tasks such as segmentation, classification and image retrieval. Many different texture representations have been proposed [1-7]. In the structural approach, texture is described by a set basic elements (shapes) and the placement rules that organize them. In statistical approaches texture is often represented, as a vector of statistical measures where these are chosen to correlate with perceived features such as: granularity, repetitiveness, directionality, etc [26].

Colour is also an important visual cue. Colour has a long and distinguished history and it is now accepted that colour is an intrinsically 3 dimensional phenomena. Each colour, viewed in a given context, can be described by three factors: hue, saturation and lightness. Importantly these factors can be related to physical measurements and so can be used to model our vision system [8].

For the most part, colour and texture have been studied as separate subjects. Yet the majority of textures that appear in the natural world have both a colour and texture aspect. So, it would make sense to investigate colour and texture together. In this paper we investigate colour-texture in the context of the human visual system.

It has long been argued that the human visual system codes images in two channels, one that carries luminance information and the other that carries chromatic information

[9]. Given this partition it is reasonable to ask whether each channel contributes to different visual tasks. For example, a study by Ramachandran [10] suggested that human perception is almost completely blind to the colour of a moving object. More recently, Livingstone et al [11,12] have also suggested that colour has minimal input into a range of preattentive visual tasks including shape from shading, illusionary contours, monocular perspective and stereopsis. McIlhagga et al [13] used low spatial frequency texture primitives to investigate the sensitivity of human preattentive texture discrimination by varying the combination of luminance and chromatic contrast and found little difference between the perception of luminance or chromatic textures. Yet, all of these studies investigate what might be characterised as 'fast' visual processing. It is well known that colour vision has a slower temporal response and so might be predicted to play a small part in 'fast' vision.

However, colour is an important cue for recognition [14]. This importance is borne out in many contemporary computer vision systems which use colour to aid recognition. For instance, Swain and Ballard [15] developed a colour indexing system, which matches images based on the similarity of colour histograms. So successful has their technique been that it is now incorporated in many imaging systems e.g. [18-21] and IBM's QBIC: Query by image content [16]. But what is the relationship between colour and texture and how might each be used in visual processing? Is there a standard colour texture representation in the same way that we have a standard colour space, or is colour texture a more malleable concept which depends on visual task or observer? Or perhaps colour and texture are completely separable; an idea supported by recent psychophysical experiments [22]. In this paper we set forth some very simple colour-texture similarity experiments. The results of these provide some insights and some possible answers to these questions.

In our experiments observers are shown two colour textures and are asked to judge their similarity. This is encoded as a number from 0 to 100 (the latter correlates with 100% similarity). Thirty-two textures were used in the experiment and all pairs were presented to each observer. The whole set of similarity judgements were placed in an observer distance matrix. Each distance matrix was analysed using the tool of Classical Multidimensional scaling [24](or CMDS). Here, each similarity is interpreted as a Euclidean distance between points in some k-dimensional space. CMDS finds a configuration of points such that the 'interpoint' straight line distances best correlates with all the similarities recorded in the similarity matrix.

A simple analysis of our data leads us to the conclusion that colour and texture combine together for some observers but are adjudged separately by others. Many of our textures share similar backgrounds and so, as one might expect, some observers group these together. Yet, many textures are coloured using different colour palettes and so it is possible that the colour information might be discounted and matching would be pattern driven. Indeed, this second type of pattern matching was also carried out. Interestingly, this latter type of matching was used by a textile designer who took part in our study. He explained his results by pointing out that a basic texture (or design) can be coloured different ways to meet the current years (fashion) colour palette or the wishes of the buyer and so colour is important to the consumer but not to the designer. That this is so, is of significant interest since colour and texture are sometimes studied together within the context of the textile industry [17].

In section 2 the psychophysical experiment is discussed. Section 3 presents some initial data resulting from a Multiscale dimensional analysis.

2 The Experiment

Selection of stimuli (colour pattern) We used 32 colour textures (or colour patterns) selected from the textile design book of David Evans Ltd, which have wide range of colour and texture variation. We scan the colour patterns and apply an industrial textile design CAD system (developed by Nedgraphics Print Ltd). Figure 1 shows the 32 colour patterns tested. The selected patterns capture a variety of different patterns such as different scales and motifs and different colourings. Some colour patterns have the same patterns with different colourways such as patterns No1-4 and patterns No 28-31.

The Observers Twelve observers participated in the study. They were selected from a range of backgrounds. The majority consisted of people with technical (engineering/computer science) backgrounds. A subset of these had substantial colour expertise and so represent an audience for whom colour is important. One observer is a professional designer for the textile industry. Non-technical (completely) naïve observers are also represented in our set of observers. None of the observers were colour blind.

Similarity Assessment Each observer was presented, in a random order, with all 496 possible pairs of stimuli (32 patterns choose 2). For each pair, the observers were asked to rate the degree of overall similarity on a scale ranging from 0 for "very dissimilar" to 100 for "very similar". There were no instructions concerning the knowledge of the attributes of the stimuli to be scaled. Each pair was shown on the same uncalibrated monitor. The order of paired comparison was randomly displayed and was different for each observer.

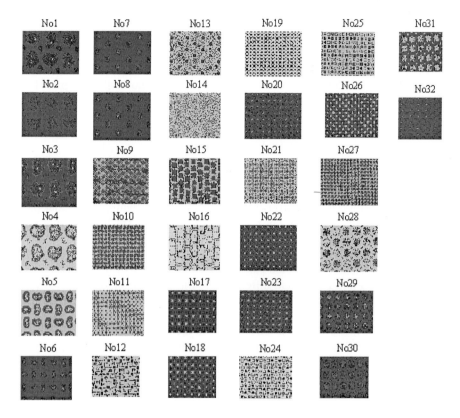

Figure 1. 32 colour patterns

3   Data analysis

Observers similarity judgements were placed in a 32x32 distance matrix $\boldsymbol{D}$. The ijth entry, $\boldsymbol{D}_{ij}$, reports the observed similarity between the ith and jth texture. By definition the distance matrix is symmetric The distance matrix for each observer is the input to classical multidimensional scaling. CMDS attempts to find a configuration of points p_i (i=1,2,...,32) such that the inter-point Euclidean distances match the similarity scores:

$$\left\| \underline{p}_i - \underline{p}_j \right\| \approx D_{ij}$$

Each point may be embedded in 2, 3 or higher dimensional space where the dimension used is a user-defined input to CMDS. Obviously the higher the dimension then the better the approximation there will be between the Euclidean distance between configuration points and the similarities in the distance matrix. Indeed, if a 32-dimensional space were used (the number of colour pattern images) then the approximation would be exact. Of course, this would mean that colour and texture would be a 32-dimensional concept.

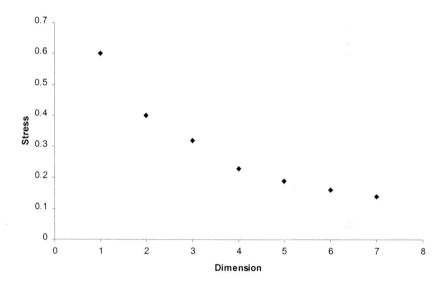

Figure 2. Stress by dimension in the tested colour texture

Obviously we would like to choose as small a dimension as possible for representing colour texture. Not only would this reflect the limited linguistic terms for colour and texture (e.g. hue and saturation and coarseness and scale) but it could ultimately lead to a compact and useful representation for consumer vision. The degree of correspondence between the distances between configuration points the distance matrix is measured by a stress function. Stress is calculated as:

$$\text{Stress} = \sqrt{\frac{\sum\sum(\|\underline{p}_i - \underline{p}_j\| - D_{ij})^2}{\sum\sum D_{ij}^2}} \qquad (1)$$

In the equation, scale refers to a constant scaling factor to keep individual stress·values between 0 and 1. When the MDS models the distance matrix exactly then the stress is zero. In general the smaller the stress, the better the representation. To find out the dimension required to represent our experimental results we compute the stress for several choices of dimension. In Figure 2 we plot average stress against dimension (for the average of 20 distance matrices from observers). It is clear that the stress diminishes as the dimension increases. Theoretically the "elbow" of the curve can be used as a guide to the dimensionality of the data. In practice determining the elbow, as demonstrated in Figure 2, is not always easy. However, perhaps 4 or 5 dimensions suffice to represent our dataset.

It is useful at this stage to interpret what stress actually means. Average stress is really a measure of the percentage of the variance in the data that is not accounted for by the configuration points. Thus, choosing 4 dimensions has a stress of 0.22 and so leaves 22% of the data unaccounted for. Even although 22% error seems large for the size of our data set is actually indicative of reasonable performance for our small dataset [25].

However, in the context of this paper we will only consider a 2-dimensional representation of colour and texture. A 2-dimensional CMDS results in 0.4 stress or 40% error and so 2 dimensions does not account for our data. However, a 2-dimensional fit is useful. Not only does it assign a 2D point to each colour texture and so allow us to plot colour textures as they appear in relation to one another. But, as we shall see, a 2-dimensional plot also allows us to qualitatively examine the similarity assessment of different observers and the relative weight that they assign to colour and texture. A more thorough quantitative analysis of higher dimensional data will follow in future work.

In Figure 3 we plot the 2-dimensional configuration points for observer DH in our study. It is clear that colour was an important cue for this observer. The three basic background colours (white gold and blue) are clustered separately. However within the individual clusters the same pattern 'factors' manifest themselves. The clusters are ordered according to scale and detail. Observer DH is representative of the similarity assessment for the majority of our observers.

In Figure 4 the configuration points for observer CR are shown. Here colour is almost irrelevant. Pattern similarity is the strongest cue. Two colour textures that differ completely in colouring but which have the same pattern are judged very similar. Conversely different patterns with the same colours are judged very different. Observer CR is a professional designer of textiles. He explained his own results by pointing out that from the designer's point of view a texture or pattern is colourless. It is something that is coloured according to the needs of a buyer or according the particular colours found in a fashion palette. This result is important since the textile industry has large image data sets (of their design industry) and they seek methods for indexing these archives.

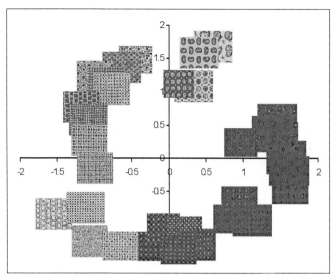

Figure 3. 2D-configuration points from observer DH

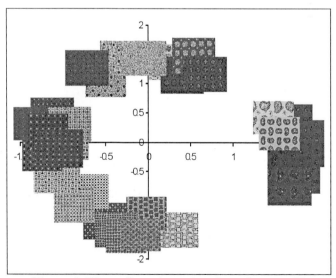

Figure 4. 2D-configuration points from observer CR

In Figure 5 the configuration points for naïve observer BT are shown. These points are somewhere in between those of DH and CR. Texture similarity here appears to be a more complex function where colour and texture are both important but which both interact with each other in an interesting way. Significantly, observer BT was a naïve observer with no background in colour, texture or imaging.

From Figures 3 through 5 we draw one conclusion: different people assess colour texture similarity differently. There are two possible explanations of this. First, is that in carrying out the similarity assessments different tasks were (implicitly) being performed. This is definitely true for the designer CR who assessed the textures in exactly the same way that he assesses designs in his day to day work. The second possibility is that each person has an intrinsically different way of assessing colour texture. Possible explanations for why this might be so include cultural differences or differences in the visual diet of the observer.

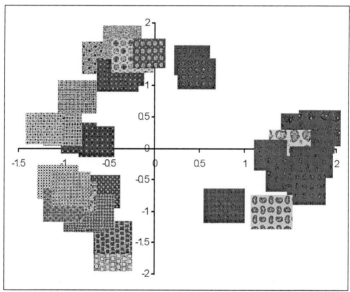

Figure 5. 2D-configuration points from observer BT

Of course if colour texture assessment is task dependent then this has implications for computer vision. For example, in the textile industry, from the designer's viewpoint, there seems little benefit in using colour in indexing applications. For other observers, colour is important but different observers judge colour texture similarity differently. If this could be explained by cultural differences then this would imply that image search engines should differ across cultures. If the differences are of a more individual nature then perhaps image search engines need to learn the colour texture features used by the individuals themselves.

4   Conclusions and further work

Based on the psychological study, colour does appear to be an important cue for colour-texture similarity for most observers. However, we found that the interactions of colour-texture strongly depend on observer. For the particular case of a textile designer colour played almost no role whatsoever. This reflects the design freedom a designer has to recolour a design in any which way the market dictates.

That individual's colour texture representations differ from one another surely has important implications for image based applications. In searching for images it is entirely probable that different people have different intrinsic notions of similarity and these depend on the visual task at hand. It follows that if automated methods seek either to replicate or assist human observers that a flexible approach needs to be taken.

In general, trading off accuracy and computation, colour and texture can be measured separately. To analyse complex colour texture accurately such as complex pattern with wide colour variation, colour and texture shouldn't be measured separately only. The interaction of colour and texture should be measured. More experiments for different applications will be conducted in the near future.

5   Acknowledgements

This work was funded by EPSRC grant GR/L60852) (Colour and Texture Selective Indexing). The authors thank all the observers for participating in the experiments. Particular thanks go to Darren Howe of Nedgraphics Print Ltd, Michael Cunha of Silk Industries Plc and Chris Roberts of Adamleys.

References

1. Brodatz P., *Textures: A photographic album for artists and designers*, Dover Publications, New York, 1966.
2. Haralick R. M., Statistical and structural approaches to texture, *Proc. of IEEE*, Vol. 67, No.5, (1979), pp.786-804.
3. Julesz B. and Bergen J. R., Textons, the fundamental elements in preattentive vision and perception of textures, *Bell System Tech.*, Vol. 62, (1983), pp.1619-1645.
4. Malik J. and Perona P., Preattentive texture discrimination with early vision mechanisms, *J. of the Optical Society of America*, Vol. 7, (1990), pp.923-932.

5. Ohanian P. P. and Dubes R. C., Performance evaluation for four classes of textural features, *Pattern Recognition*, Vol. 25 (1992) pp.819-833.
6. Rao R. and Lohse G. L., Towards a texture naming systems: identifying relevant dimensions of texture perception, *IBM Research Technical Report*, NO. RC 19140 (1993).
7. Rao R. and Lohse G. L., Towards a texture naming system: Identifying relevant dimensions of texture, *Vision Research*, Vol. 36, No. 11, (1996), pp.1649-1669.
8. Hunt R. W. G., *The Reproduction of Colour*, 5th Edition, Fountain Press, (1995).
9. Schacter B. J., Davis L. S. and Rosenfeld A., Scene segmentation by cluster detection in color space, *Technical Report*, Computer Science Center, University of Maryland, (1975).
10. Ramachandran V. S., Does colour provide an input to human motion perception? *Nature*, Vol. 275, (1978), pp.55-56.
11. Livingston M. S. and Huber D., Psychophysical evidence for separate channels for the perception of the form, colour, movement and depth, *J. Neuroscience*, 7 (1987) pp.3416-3468.
12. Livingston M. S. and Huber D., Segregation of form, colour, movement and depth: anatomy, *Physiology and Perception, Science*, Vol. 240, (1987), pp.740-749.
13. McIlhagga W., Hine T., Cole G. R. and Snyder A. W., Texture segregation with luminance and chromatic contrast, *Vision Research*, Vol. 30, No. 3, (1990), pp. 489-495.
14. Wurm L. and Legge G. E., Color improved object recognition in normal and low vision, *J. of Exp. Psych.*, 19(4), (1993), pp.899-911.
15. Swain M. J. and Ballard D. H., Colour indexing, *International Journal of Computer Vision*, Vol. 7, No. 1, (1991), pp.11-32.
16. Flickner M., Sawhney H., Niblack W., Ashley J., Huang Q., Dom B., Gorkani M., Hafner J., Lee D., Petkovic D., Steele D., and Yanker P., Query by image and video content - the QBIC system, *Computer*, Vol. 28, No. 9, (1995), pp.23-32.
17. Niblack W., Zhu X., and Hafner J., Updates to the QBIC system, *SPIE Proceedings* (1997), Vol. 3312, pp.150-161.
18. Stricker M. and Orengo M., Similarity of color images, *SPIE*, Vol. 2420, No. 1, (1995), Vol. 2420, pp.381-392.
19. Paschos G., Chromatic correlation features for texture recognition, *Pattern Recognition Letters*, Vol. 19, (1998), pp.643-650.
20. Jain A. and Healey G., A multiscale representation including opponent color features for texture recognition, *IEEE Transactions on Image Processing*, Vol. 7, No.1, (1998), pp.124-128.
21. Finlayson G. D. and Tian G. Y., Colour indexing across illumination, *The Proceedings of Content-Based Image Retrieval*, Newcastle, 1999.

22. Poirson B. and Wandell B. A., Appearance of colored patterns: pattern-color separability, *J. Opt. Soc. Am. A*, Vol. 10, No.12, (1993), pp.2458-2470.
23. Poirson B. and Wandell B. A., Pattern-color separable pathways predict sensitivity to simple colored patterns, *Vision Research*, Vol. 36, No. 4, (1996), pp.515-526.
24. Schiffman S. S., Reynolds M. L. and Young F. W., *Introduction to multidimensional scaling*, Academic Press, New York, 1981.
25. Young F. W. and Hamer R. M., *Theory and Applications of Multidimensional Scaling*, Eribaum Associates, Hillsdale, NJ, 1994.
26. Liu F. and Picard R. W., Periodicity, directionality, and randomness: wold features for image modeling and retrieval, *IEEE Trans. on PAMI*, Vol. 18, No.7, (1996), pp.722-733.

MULTISPECTRAL TEXTURE DERIVATION IN VIRTUAL COLORING

V. BOTCHKO

Department of Information Technology, Lappeenranta University of Technology,
P.O. Box 20, FIN-53851 Lappeenranta, Finland
E-mail: Vladimir.Botchko@lut.fi

S. NAKAUCHI

Department of Information and Computer Sciences,
Toyohashi University of Technology, Hibarigaoka Tempaku Toyohashi 441-8580,
Japan
E-mail: naka@bpel.tutics.tut.ac.jp

J. PARKKINEN

Department of Computer Science, University of Joensuu, P.O. Box 111,
FIN-80101 Joensuu, Finland
E-mail: Jussi.Parkkinen@cs.joensuu.fi

H. KÄLVIÄINEN

Department of Information Technology, Lappeenranta University of Technology,
P.O. Box 20, FIN-53851 Lappeenranta, Finland
E-mail: Heikki.Kalviainen@lut.fi

In this paper, a virtual coloring technique for texture images is described. This technique is important in multispectral image research investigating the relationship between color and texture information in the image. At least low order statistics are needed to define color when color texture is represented by color reproduction in a multispectral image. In the spectral domain, the mean spectrum and spectrum standard deviation are needed for virtual spectral color reproduction. The properties of multispectral texture images and their derivation in virtual coloring are discussed. It is shown how the color changes in texture. This approach can also be used for object transparency simulation. A stochastic model for color texture reproduction and experimental results are given.

1 Introduction

Coloring techniques for gray level pictures or images are needed in different areas of computer graphics. In many cases pseudocolor or false color techniques are used.[1-5] A pseudocolor image is usually considered a color image produced from a monochrome image. A false color image is a modified color image from an original natural color image or from multispectral image com-

113

ponents. In the synthesis of photorealistic images, e.g. for virtual environments or in movie animation, natural coloring is added to artificial scenes.[6,7] In this paper, we describe a method for producing naturally colored texture images.

The basic principle of our approach is to produce a multicomponent image from a given gray level texture image and, then, to produce a color image from the multicomponent image. The multicomponent image can be produced based on multispectral texture properties. Since, these colors are artificially produced and model natural color spectra, we call them virtual colors. The colors are based on a realistic spectrum reconstruction model. This differs from traditional coloring in RGB space. The approach keeps the realistic relationship between color and texture and the model parameters are derived from multispectral images of natural scenes. This virtual color approach can be considered novel.

A number of methods for multispectral texture modeling and analysis have been proposed. The Markov random field texture model and the statistical approach for a color image using correlation functions defined within and between components were proposed by Healey and Wang.[8] A variety of techniques have been used to synthesize multispectral texture. Multispectral extensions of the simultaneous autoregressive and Markov random field models were developed, based on the RGB color model.[9] These models are effective at capturing the essential characteristics of natural textures, but they are restricted in natural color modeling.

The proposed virtual color technique deals with a multicomponent image that allows us to use the spectral characteristics of the natural objects and to get photorealistic image coloring. Spectra and gray level textures can be acquired in different places and at different times, although they must correspond to one another. The technique presented is based on a recent study by the authors.[10,11]

In this paper, our aim is to show that the spectral color representation gives a good basis for photorealistic coloring of artificially colored images. Best results are obtained, when the mean and standard deviation of the color are considered as vectors based on the color spectrum.

In Sec. 2, we describe the image model for a color image with a n-dimensional vector representing the color of each pixel. In Sec. 3, the model parameters are studied based on spectral images from a natural scene and, in Sec. 4, the algorithm for production of a virtual color image based on a gray level texture image is given. Sec. 5 describes tests for virtual coloring and applications of the approach are discussed in Sec. 6.

2 Image model

Let us first consider the multispectral statistical image model. A multi-spectral texture image is composed of a set of images at different optical wavelengths and can be presented by a n-dimensional vector random field $\boldsymbol{\nu}(\boldsymbol{x}) = (\nu_1(\boldsymbol{x}), \nu_2(\boldsymbol{x}), \ldots, \nu_n(\boldsymbol{x}))^T$, where the vector $\boldsymbol{x} = (x_1, x_2)^T$, x_1, x_2 are the spatial dimensions, $1, 2, \ldots, n$ are indices of the spectral dimension, and T denotes the transpose. Each element of $\boldsymbol{\nu}(\boldsymbol{x})$ in the spatial domain can be described in terms of the mean component and the fluctuation component. This corresponds to one ton-texture concept.[12] Hence, the field $\boldsymbol{\nu}(\boldsymbol{x})$ is characterized

$$\boldsymbol{\nu}(\boldsymbol{x}) = \boldsymbol{\mu} + \boldsymbol{D}\,\boldsymbol{\eta}(\boldsymbol{x}) \tag{1}$$

where $\boldsymbol{\mu}$ is a mean vector $\boldsymbol{\mu} = (\mu_1, \ldots, \mu_n)^T$, $\boldsymbol{D}$ is a diagonal matrix $\boldsymbol{D} = diag(\sigma_1, \sigma_2, \ldots, \sigma_n)$, and $\boldsymbol{\sigma}$ is a standard deviation vector $\boldsymbol{\sigma} = (\sigma_1, \sigma_2, \ldots, \sigma_n)^T$, $\boldsymbol{\eta}(\boldsymbol{x})$ is a vector random field with zero mean and unit standard deviation for each component $\boldsymbol{\eta}(\boldsymbol{x}) = (\eta_1(\boldsymbol{x}), \eta_2(\boldsymbol{x}), \ldots, \eta_n(\boldsymbol{x}))^T$. The vector $\boldsymbol{\eta}(\boldsymbol{x})$ contains the correlated component fields.

Next, the stochastic properties of a fluctuation component are considered. The following discussion is based on the separability assumption for the spectral and spatial components of the covariance matrix.[13] This assumption allows the covariance matrix to be presented as the Kronecker matrix product of the spatial and spectral covariance matrices

$$\boldsymbol{K}_\nu = \begin{pmatrix} k_{11}\sigma_1^2\boldsymbol{K}_\eta & k_{12}\sigma_1\sigma_2\boldsymbol{K}_\eta & \ldots & k_{1n}\sigma_1\sigma_n\boldsymbol{K}_\eta \\ k_{21}\sigma_2\sigma_1\boldsymbol{K}_\eta & k_{22}\sigma_2^2\boldsymbol{K}_\eta & \ldots & k_{2n}\sigma_2\sigma_n\boldsymbol{K}_\eta \\ \vdots & \vdots & \vdots & \vdots \\ k_{n1}\sigma_n\sigma_1\boldsymbol{K}_\eta & k_{n2}\sigma_n\sigma_2\boldsymbol{K}_\eta & \ldots & k_{nn}\sigma_n^2\boldsymbol{K}_\eta \end{pmatrix} \tag{2}$$

where $\boldsymbol{K}_\eta$ is a Toeplitz-block Toeplitz matrix of a random field component (the component of $\boldsymbol{\eta}(\boldsymbol{x})$) mapped into a vector by column (or row) ordering, k_{ij} is the (i, j) element of the covariance matrix $\boldsymbol{K}$ and describes the correlation between any pixel pairs.

We assume that the matrix $\boldsymbol{K}$ is the covariance matrix of the first-order stationary Markov sequence. Hence, the covariance matrix $\boldsymbol{K}$ can be presented as

$$\boldsymbol{K} = \begin{pmatrix} 1 & \rho & \ldots & \rho^{n-1} \\ \rho & 1 & \ldots & \rho^{n-2} \\ \vdots & \vdots & \vdots & \vdots \\ \rho^{n-1} & \rho^{n-2} & \ldots & 1 \end{pmatrix} \tag{3}$$

where ρ is a correlation coefficient.

3   Statistical Analysis of Natural Images

To produce test images in virtual coloring, we analyzed a set of natural images and derived parameters for the model. An imaging spectrometer, ImSpector, was used for the experimental study. The spectral line camera provided 384-pixel spatial information of a line image and 286 discrete wavelengths in the range from 401.5 nm to 716.5 nm, with 1.1 nm resolution. To get the full two-dimensional image, the camera was placed on a table which was moved in a horizontal direction to provide the other spatial dimension, with an image size of 95-105 lines. A few multispectral images of flowers outdoors were acquired. They were obtained with sun illumination.

If we consider the basic properties of multispectral images, according to the multispectral statistical image model, low order statistics: the initial first and central second moments (mean vector, standard deviation vector and correlation coefficient) are the most important color definition factors. Therefore, we investigated them in the real multispectral images. The regions in each image which could be examined visually as texture were selected. The regions had different colors. The results showed that all the tested color regions had the values of the standard deviation vector components approximately proportional to the values of the mean spectrum components (Fig. 1). The mean (solid line) and standard deviation (dashed line) vectors for the texture regions $a - h$ with the different colors are shown in Fig. 1 $a - h$, respectively. Color reproduction of the multispectral test image for the marked regions $a - h$ is shown in Fig. 5.

The correlation coefficient was measured between each two components separated by an interval 5.5 nm. It is in agreement with spectral resolution of the imaging spectrometer which is 5 nm according to the Rayleigh criterion. The correlation coefficient for the regions b (red roses) and g (green leaves) is shown in Fig. 2 and Fig. 3, respectively. First, it can be noticed that the correlation coefficient is almost constant and close to one in a wide subrange of wavelengths. However, it decreases for some wavelengths. There are two reasons for this. The decrease in the far blue region (the short wavelength subregion) can be explained by the noise of the spectral camera. In the blue region, the spectral camera sensitivity is small and the effect of decorrelated noise increases. At the ends of the approximately constant coefficient regions, the correlation coefficient decreases due to image statistic change. In this study, we neglect this effect and consider the correlation coefficient constant.

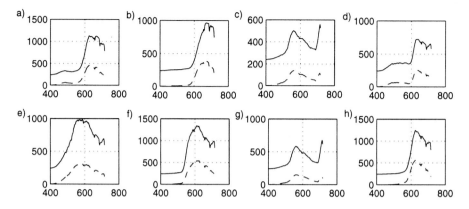

Figure 1. The mean (solid line) and standard deviation (dashed line) vector elements for the color texture regions $a - h$ marked in Fig. 5. The x-axis is the wavelength, and the y-axis is the pixel value.

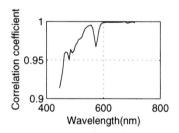

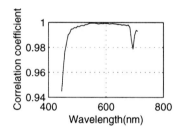

Figure 2. Correlation coefficient for region b (red roses).

Figure 3. Correlation coefficient for region g (green leaves).

We, nevertheless, expect to keep quality image coloring.

4 Texture Coloring Algorithm

Obviously, the vector $\boldsymbol{\mu}$ defines color properties in the case of color homogeneous regions. For texture regions, the fluctuation component has to be taken into account to ascertain how texture affects color reproduction through the multispectral image. This texture factor plays no less an important role in color image reproduction than the mean component and it is used in the coloring algorithm.

In coloring, first a multicomponent image is produced from a given gray level image. Then, a color image is produced from a multicomponent image. Hence, the gray level image and a spectrum are given. To get the elements of μ the given spectrum is sampled at equal intervals. Then, each sample is an element of μ.

The fluctuation component can be defined from parameters ρ, σ, K_η according to Eq. 2 . If a gray level texture image is given K_η is determined. The gray level texture image coloring technique requires the image data to be normalized, i.e. to have the mean zero and the standard deviation equal to one. This simulates an element of a vector field $\eta(x)$.

Next, a normalized gray level image has to be copied several times to provide a vector field $\eta(x)$. This corresponds to the situation when each element of matrix K is equal to one ($\rho = 1$).

It was shown in Sec. 3 that the vector σ elements are approximately proportional to the corresponding elements of μ. Hence, the standard deviation vector can be characterized

$$\sigma = \beta(\mu - \mu_{min}) \tag{4}$$

where β is a proportional coefficient $0 \leq \beta < 1$, μ_{min} is a column vector with all the elements equal to the minimum value of μ and the same size as μ. Condition $\rho = 1$ and operation $(\mu - \mu_{min})$ lead to a singular covariance matrix. However, computation with a covariance matrix is not used in this approach.

For generalization, the standard deviation vector is presented as follows

$$\sigma = \alpha\beta(\mu - \mu_{min}) + (1 - \alpha)c\varepsilon \tag{5}$$

where α is a weight coefficient $0 \leq \alpha \leq 1$, c is a constant, ε is a column vector with all the unity elements and the same size as μ.

Finally, Eq. 1 is computed. As a result, each gray level pixel has its own specific spectrum and can be reproduced as a color pixel. For reproduction, a convenient color system is used.

Thus, the gray level texture coloring algorithm is as follows

1. Normalize the original image.

2. Copy the normalized image n times to get a vector field $\boldsymbol{\eta}(\boldsymbol{x})$ (n is the number of spectral channels).

3. Set the mean vector $\boldsymbol{\mu}$ equal to the given sampled spectrum $\boldsymbol{s}$.

4. Set the standard deviation vector $\boldsymbol{\sigma}$: $\boldsymbol{\sigma} = \alpha\beta(\boldsymbol{\mu} - \boldsymbol{\mu}_{min}) + (1 - \alpha)c\boldsymbol{\varepsilon}$.

5. Compute the vector field $\boldsymbol{\nu}(\boldsymbol{x})$: $\boldsymbol{\nu}(\boldsymbol{x}) = \boldsymbol{\mu} + \boldsymbol{D}\,\boldsymbol{\eta}(\boldsymbol{x})$.

6. Reproduce a multicomponent image in a suitable color system (e.g. RGB CIE 1931).

7. Enhance texture contrast by increasing the fluctuation component if necessary (increase β and go to Step 4).

5 Virtual Coloring

In this section the virtual color technique, which is very simple in implementation and useful in producing photorealistic color images from the gray level texture images, is considered. The texture images and spectra can be taken from any database. The spectra for virtual coloring can be arbitrary given by the designer or the color can be produced from its spectral characteristics.

5.1 Virtual Color Image Tests with Brodatz Texture and Munsell Spectra

First an experiment was conducted with gray level textures. Four texture images from the Brodatz texture album, shown in Fig. 7, were taken.[14] The parts of these images with size 128×128 were used. From left to right their album numbers are 3, 28, 57, 77.

The result of virtual coloring by using the spectra from the color spectrum database[15] is presented in Fig. 8. The spectra were measured from the color samples in the Munsell Book of Color.[16] The spectra correspond to the Munsell samples with Munsell Notation, i.e. $2.5YV7C10$ (yellow (Y), Hue 2.5, Value 7, Chroma 10). This is shown in Table 1. The virtual texture coloring with a small color difference is shown in Fig. 6 and the corresponding Munsell Notation is given in Table 2. It is possible to notice the color change after coloring. The color of the light part of texture has the desired color used in coloring. The shadow part has color with an opposite shift from the mean

Table 1. Data for Fig. 8

Brodatz texture number Munsell sample number Munsell Notation			
3	28	57	77
588	116	364	1162
$2.5YV7C10$	$10GYV5C8$	$2.5BV5C8$	$7.5RV4C12$

Table 2. Data for Fig. 6

Brodatz texture number Munsell sample number Munsell Notation			
3	28	57	77
591	114	362	1156
$2.5YV8.5C10$	$10GYV7C8$	$2.5BV7C8$	$7.5RV7C10$
3	28	57	77
587	115	363	1161
$2.5YV8C10$	$10GYV6C8$	$2.5BV6C8$	$7.5RV5C12$
3	28	57	77
588	116	364	1162
$2.5YV7C10$	$10GYV5C8$	$2.5BV5C8$	$7.5RV4C12$

according to Eq. 1. Such an effect can be found in the case of high texture contrast. In the case of low contrast, the shadow part will have a tendency to get the opponent color shift. This opponent color shift effect will be more clearly demonstrated in Subsec. 5.2.

5.2 Virtual Coloring Using Spectral Characteristics

According to the multispectral statistical image model, the low order statistics are the most important color definition factors. If the correlation coefficient is assumed to be a constant, then only two factors need to be considered. They are the mean vector μ and the standard deviation vector σ.

First, virtual coloring with a constant mean spectrum was used. This is shown in Fig. 9. This result confirms the previous conclusion that pixels with spectrum values greater than the mean spectrum have a more saturated color than pixels with the mean spectrum. The pixels with spectrum values less than the mean spectrum have the opposite color shift than the color reproduced by the mean spectrum. With the exception of μ, the four colored images presented in Fig. 9 all have the same parameters as the images shown in Fig. 8. Thus, Fig. 9 shows how the color changes in texture or in the fluctuation component.

Next, the standard deviation was fixed (the standard deviation vector elements are constant) and the mean spectrum was unfixed. The results are shown in Fig. 10. With the exception of σ, the four colored images presented in Fig. 10 all have the same parameters as the images shown in Fig. 8. Basically, color is represented here by saturation change. And it is close to the pseudocoloring technique. This kind of coloring is widely used in cartographic data mapping and many graphics editors.

Using the generalized model Eq. 5, one can get the intermediate results by computing the weighted sum of the variable and constant components of σ. This is shown in Fig. 11. For Fig. 11 from left to right $\alpha = 1, \alpha = 0.8, \alpha = 0.5, \alpha = 0$, respectively.

5.3 Virtual Coloring of Composed Image

In this section the virtual coloring algorithm for the composed images is discussed. The composed image and spectra for coloring are given. An aerial image of a forest fire acquired in the St. Petersburg region (Russia) on July of 1995 was used. As spectrum for the virtual coloring of the forest region we used real spectra measured from spruce and birch forest.[15,17]

The original RGB color image is presented in Fig. 12. This image was converted into a gray level image shown in Fig. 4. Next, the image was segmented into forest, smoke and overlapping regions.[18–20]

First, the smoke and the forest regions were segmented. Then, the smoke region was partitioned into a central and border part. The results of the texture segmentation are presented in Fig. 4. The central smoke region spectrum was artificially modeled. We produced both a spruce and birch color version of the forest, as explained in Subsec. 5.1. The spruce and birch spectra were taken from a database [15] and used for forest coloring in Fig. 13 and Fig. 14, respectively. Then, for the border region the optical transparency model was used. The additive model[21] for a mixed spectrum is presented by

$$s = \gamma s_f + (1 - \gamma)s_s \tag{6}$$

where s_f is a forest spectrum from the database, s_s is a smoke artificial spectrum, γ is a weight coefficient $0 \leq \gamma \leq 1$.

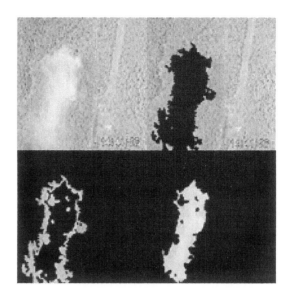

Figure 4. The converted gray level image (upper left) and the results of segmentation.

The virtual color image (spruce spectrum) with $\gamma = 0.4$ is presented in Fig. 13 and the virtual color image (birch spectrum) with $\gamma = 0.55$ is presented in Fig. 14. The result seems to be relatively good.

6 Discussion

In this paper a novel approach, called virtual coloring, for photorealistic color texture reproduction is presented. Virtual coloring is based on the use of color spectra for the color representation. An advantage of the use of spectra is the production of more realistic and, in some cases, more accurate colors.

This method can be applied to real world scene reproduction, e.g. in computer graphics, and cartographic applications. By combining the estimation of the spectral characteristics, the virtual coloring can also be used in multispectral image compression-decompression.

The color can be defined by using real measured spectra or it can be reconstructed from its spectral characteristics. In Fig. 13 and Fig. 14 an example of virtual coloring of a frame from an airborne color video is given. When compared to the real color image of the frame (Fig. 12), one can see the usability of the method.

Acknowledgments

The aerial image of a forest fire was obtained from the Research Institute Prognoz at St. Petersburg Electrotechnical University, St. Petersburg, Russia.

References

1. A. P. Krishna, Land Cover Change Dynamics of a Himalayan Watershed Utilizing Indian Remote Sensing Satellite (IRS) Data, *Proc. International Geoscience and Remote Sensing Symposium, IGARSS'96*, Vol. 1, 1996, Lincoln, NE, US, pp. 221-223.
2. T. M. Lehmann, A. Kaser, R. Repges, A Simple Parametric Equation for Pseudocoloring Grey Scale Images Keeping Their Original Brightness Progression, *Image and Vision Computing*, Vol. 15, No. 3, 1997, pp. 251-257.
3. C. Ware, Color Sequences for Univariate Maps: Theory, Experiments and Principles, *IEEE Computer Graphics and Applications*, Vol. 8, No. 5 , Sept., 1988, pp. 41 -49.
4. A. K. Jain, *Fundamentals of Digital Image Processing*, Prentice Hall, NJ, 1989.
5. W. K. Pratt, *Digital Image Processing*, John Wiley & Sons, NY, 1991.
6. J. D. Foley, A. van Dam, S. K. Feiner, J. F. Hughes, *Computer Graphics: Principles and Practice*, Addison-Wesley, MA, 1990.
7. R. Freidhoff, W. Benzon, *Visualization: the Second Computer Revolution*, Harry N. Abrams, NY, 1989.
8. G. Healey and L. Wang, Illumination-Invariant Recognition of Texture in Color Images, *J. Opt. Soc. Am.*, Vol. A12, No. 9, Sept. 1995, pp. 1877-1883.
9. J. Bennett and A. Khotanzad, Multispectral Random Field Models for Synthesis and Analysis of Color Images, *IEEE Trans. Pattern Anal. Machine Intell. (PAMI)*, Vol. PAMI-20, No. 3, March, 1998, pp. 327-332.
10. V. Botchko, J. Auvinen, O. Mäkinen,, J. Parkkinen, H. Kälviäinen, Parametric Multispectral Texture Modeling, *Proc. Scandinavian Conference on Image Analysis, SCIA'99*, June 7-11, 1999, Kangerlussuaq, Greenland, pp. 763-769.
11. V. Botchko, S. Nakauchi, J. Parkkinen, H. Kälviäinen, Virtual Coloring of Texture, *Proc. Workshop on Texture Analysis in Machine Vision, TEXTURE'99*, June 14-15, 1999, Oulu, Finland, pp. 165-171.

12. R. M. Haralick, Statistical and Structural Approaches to Texture, *Proc. of the IEEE,* Vol. 67, 1979, pp. 786-804.

13. B. R. Hunt, O. Kübler, Karhunen-Loeve Multispectral Image Restoration, Part I: Theory, *IEEE Trans. Acoust., Speech, and Signal Processing,* Vol. 32, No. 3, June, 1984, pp. 592-600.

14. P. Brodatz, *Textures: A Photographic Album for Artists and Designers,* Dover Publications, NY, 1966.

15. *www.it.lut.fi/research/color/lutcs_database.html*

16. *Munsell Book of Color, Matte Finish Collection,* (Munsell Color, Baltimore, 1976).

17. R. Silvennoinen, T. Jaaskelainen, K. Nygren, J. Hiltunen, J. Parkkinen, Temporal, Spatial and Environmental Characteristics of Pine Reflectance Spectra, *Environmental Science and Technology,* Vol. 29, No. 6, 1995, pp. 1456-1459.

18. C. W. Therrien, T. F. Quatiery, D. E. Dudgeon, Statistical Model-Based Algorithms for Image Analysis, *Proceedings of the IEEE,* Vol. 74, No. 4, April, 1986, pp. 532-551.

19. T. S. Huang, *Two-Dimensional Digital Signal Processing II: Transforms and Median Filters,* T. S. Huang, ed., Springer-Verlag, Berlin, 1981.

20. J. Besag, On the Statistical Analysis of Dirty Pictures, *J. Royal Statist. Soc.,* Vol. 48, Ser. B, No. 3, 1986, pp. 259-302.

21. S. Nakauchi, S. Usui, J. Parkkinen, P. Silfsten, A Computational Theory of Color Transparency, *Proc. Scandinavian Conference on Image Analysis, SCIA'99,* June 7-11, 1999, Kangerlussuaq, Greenland, pp. 561-568.

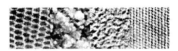

Figure 7. Brodatz texture images.

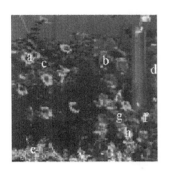

Figure 5. Test image.

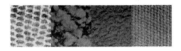

Figure 8. Texture coloring.

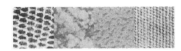

Figure 9. Texture coloring (fixed μ).

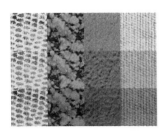

Figure 6. Coloring (small color difference).

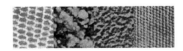

Figure 10. Texture coloring (fixed σ).

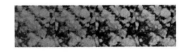

Figure 11. Coloring, $\alpha = 1$(left), $0.8, 0.5, 0$.

126

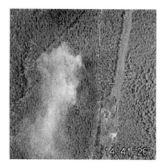

Figure 12. Color image.

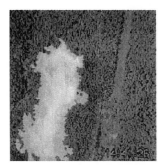

Figure 13. Coloring, spruce spectrum, $\gamma = 0.4$.

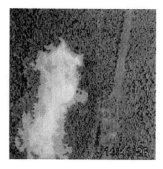

Figure 14. Coloring, birch spectrum, $\gamma = 0.55$.

APPLICATIONS

USING TEXTURE IN IMAGE SIMILARITY AND RETRIEVAL

SELIM AKSOY AND ROBERT M. HARALICK

Intelligent Systems Laboratory, Department of Electrical Engineering,
University of Washington, Seattle, WA 98195-2500, U.S.A.
E-mail: {aksoy,haralick}@isl.ee.washington.edu

Texture has been one of the most popular representations in image retrieval. Our image database retrieval system uses two sets of textural features, first one being the line-angle-ratio statistics which is a macro texture measure that uses a texture histogram computed from the spatial relationships of intersecting lines as well as the properties of their surroundings, second one being the variances of gray level spatial dependencies computed from co-occurrence matrices as micro texture measures. This paper also discusses a line selection algorithm to eliminate insignificant lines and statistical feature selection methods to select the best performing subset of features to adjust the parameters of the feature extraction algorithms. Average precision is used to evaluate the retrieval performance in comparative tests with three other texture analysis algorithms. Experiments on a database of approximately 10,000 images show that low-level textural features can help in grouping images into semantically meaningful categories and our method is fast and effective with an average precision of 0.73 when 12 images are retrieved.

1 Introduction

Texture has been one of the most important characteristics which have been used to classify and recognize objects and scenes. Haralick and Shapiro [16] defined texture as the uniformity, density, coarseness, roughness, regularity, intensity and directionality of discrete tonal features and their spatial relationships. Haralick [14] gave a review of two main approaches to characterize and measure texture: *statistical* approaches and *structural* approaches. A recent texture survey was done by Tuceryan and Jain, [30] where texture models were classified into statistical methods, geometrical methods, model-based methods and signal processing methods.

Image databases are becoming increasingly popular due to the large amount of images that are generated by various applications and the advances in computer technology. Initial work on content-based retrieval focused on using low-level features like color and texture. One of the first systems that used texture in finding similarities between images is the IBM's QBIC Project, where Flickner et al. [12] used features based on coarseness, contrast, and directionality that were proposed by Tamura et al. [29] In the MIT Photobook Project, Pentland et al. [27] used 2-D Wold-based decompositions [22] as texture descriptions. In the Los Alamos National Lab.'s CAN-

DID Project, Kelly *et al.* [19] used Laws' texture energy maps and a sum of weighted Gaussians to model the texture. Manjunath and Ma [24] used Gabor filter-based multi-resolution representations to extract texture information. Li and Castelli [20] used 21 different spatial features like gray level differences, co-occurrence matrices, moments, autocorrelation functions and fractals on remote sensing images. Smith [28] used energies of the quadrature mirror filter wavelet filter bank outputs at different resolutions as textural features. The main disadvantages of these approaches are that they are either ineffective when a large database of images with non-homogeneous textures are used, or require a lot of computation.

More recent approaches by Carson *et al.* [7] and Ma and Manjunath [23] developed region-based query systems which involve image segmentation based on color and texture but the region segmentation algorithms are still too slow to be used in an image retrieval application. Even though there have been further approaches that use post-processing methods like relevance feedback to improve retrieval accuracy, these methods still depend heavily on the feature representations and therefore it is crucial to improve the low-level feature extraction algorithms to improve overall retrieval.

In this paper we attempt to improve retrieval efficiency using easy-to-compute low-level features that combine macro and micro aspects of the texture in the image. The first set of texture features are the line-angle-ratio statistics. These are macro texture measures that use spatial relationships between lines as well as the properties of their surroundings. A statistical line selection algorithm to eliminate insignificant lines is part of the method. The second set of texture features consist of the variances of gray level spatial dependencies. These are micro texture measures that use second-order (co-occurrence) statistics of gray levels of pixels in particular spatial relationships. Both sets of features are integrated for a multi-scale texture analysis which is crucial for a compact representation, especially for large databases containing different types of complex images.

We use a two-class pattern classification approach to find statistical measures of how well some of the features perform better than others to avoid having less significant or even redundant features that increase computation but contribute very little in the decision process. Retrieval performance is evaluated using average precision computed for the manually groundtruthed data set.

The rest of the paper is organized as follows. First, the textural features are presented in Sections 2, 3 and 4. Then, feature selection methods are described in Section 5. Experiments and results are discussed in Section 6. Finally, conclusions are given in Section 7.

2   Line-Angle-Ratio Statistics

Experiments on various types of images showed us that one of the strongest spatial features of an image is its line segments. Edge and line information have been extensively used in both very early and recent approaches to texture. Our algorithm is composed of two stages; pre-processing and texture histogram generation.

2.1   Pre-processing

Each image is processed by Canny's edge detector, [6] Etemadi's edge linker, [11] a line selection operator and a line grouping operator to detect line pairs to associate with it a set of feature records. Edge detection followed by line detection often results in many false alarms. It is especially hard to select proper parameters for these operators if one does not have groundtruth information as training data. After line detection, we use hypothesis testing to eliminate lines that do not have significant difference between the gray level distributions in the regions on their right and left.

The algorithm we developed for line selection is given as follows. Let the set of N gray levels $x_1, x_2, \ldots, x_N$ be considered as iid $N(\mu_x, \sigma_x^2)$ samples from the region to the right of a line and the set of M gray levels $y_1, y_2, \ldots, y_M$ be considered as iid $N(\mu_y, \sigma_y^2)$ samples from the region to the left of that line. Define

$$\bar{x} = \frac{1}{N} \sum_{n=1}^{N} x_n \quad \sim \quad N\left(\mu_x, \frac{\sigma_x^2}{N}\right)$$

and

$$\bar{y} = \frac{1}{M} \sum_{m=1}^{M} y_m \quad \sim \quad N\left(\mu_y, \frac{\sigma_y^2}{M}\right).$$

Then the random variable $z = \bar{x} - \bar{y}$ has a distribution

$$N(\mu_z, \sigma_z^2) = N\left(\mu_x - \mu_y, \frac{\sigma_x^2}{N} + \frac{\sigma_y^2}{M}\right).$$

Define the null hypothesis as $H_0 : \mu_x = \mu_y$ and $\sigma_x = \sigma_y$ which means both sets of gray levels come from the same distribution, and the alternative hypothesis as $H_1 : \mu_x \neq \mu_y$ and $\sigma_x \neq \sigma_y$. To form the test statistic, define two random variables A and B as

$$A = \left(\frac{z - \mu_z}{\sigma_z}\right)^2 \quad \sim \quad \chi_1^2 \tag{1}$$

and

$$B = \frac{1}{N-1} \sum_{n=1}^{N} \left(\frac{x - \bar{x}}{\sigma_x} \right)^2 + \frac{1}{M-1} \sum_{m=1}^{M} \left(\frac{y - \bar{y}}{\sigma_y} \right)^2 \quad \sim \chi^2_{N+M-2}. \quad (2)$$

Then, define the test statistic $F = \frac{A/1}{B/(N+M-2)}$ which, under the null hypothesis, becomes

$$F = \frac{z^2 \frac{(N+M-2)}{(\frac{1}{N}+\frac{1}{M})}}{\frac{1}{(N-1)} \sum_{n=1}^{N}(x-\bar{x})^2 + \frac{1}{(M-1)} \sum_{m=1}^{M}(y-\bar{y})^2} \quad \sim F_{1,N+M-2}. \quad (3)$$

Given a threshold for the F-value, if the null hypothesis H_0 is true, the line is rejected, if the alternative hypothesis H_1 is true, the line is accepted as a significant one.

After obtaining relatively significant lines, we use a line grouping operator to find intersecting and/or near-intersecting line pairs. We allow near-intersection instead of exact end-point intersection because of the perturbation due to noise.

Given two lines L_1 and L_2 with end-points $(P_1, P_2) = ([r_1 \, c_1]', [r_2 \, c_2]')$ and $(P_3, P_4) = ([r_3 \, c_3]', [r_4 \, c_4]')$ respectively, equations of them can be written as

$$L_1: \quad P = P_1 + \lambda_1(P_2 - P_1), \quad (4)$$
$$L_2: \quad P = P_3 + \lambda_2(P_4 - P_3) \quad (5)$$

where λ_1 and λ_2 are real constants between 0 and 1. The following conditions should be satisfied for intersection:

$$r_1 + \lambda_1(r_2 - r_1) = r_3 + \lambda_2(r_4 - r_3), \quad (6)$$
$$c_1 + \lambda_1(c_2 - c_1) = c_3 + \lambda_2(c_4 - c_3). \quad (7)$$

If $(r_4 - r_3)(c_2 - c_1) = (r_2 - r_1)(c_4 - c_3)$, lines L_1 and L_2 are parallel. If also $(r_2 - r_1)(c_3 - c_1) = (r_3 - r_1)(c_2 - c_1)$, end-points P_1, P_2, P_3, P_4 are co-linear. If neither of these cases are true, λ_1 and λ_2 can be derived from Eq. (6) and (7) as

$$\lambda_2 = \frac{(r_2 - r_1)(c_3 - c_1) - (r_3 - r_1)(c_2 - c_1)}{(r_4 - r_3)(c_2 - c_1) - (r_2 - r_1)(c_4 - c_3)} \quad (8)$$

and

$$\lambda_1 = \frac{r_3 - r_1}{r_2 - r_1} + \lambda_2 \frac{r_4 - r_3}{r_2 - r_1} \quad \text{if } r_1 \neq r_2$$

$$\text{or} \tag{9}$$

$$= \frac{c_3 - c_1}{c_2 - c_1} + \lambda_2 \frac{c_4 - c_3}{c_2 - c_1} \quad \text{if } c_1 \neq c_2.$$

We define *Tol* as the tolerance, in number of pixels, for the end points of the lines to intersect. We need to define this tolerance to allow near-intersection instead of exact end-point intersection. To determine the tolerances for λ_1 and λ_2, two new tolerances τ_1 and τ_2 can be defined as

$$\tau_1 = \frac{Tol}{||P_2 P_1||} \quad \text{and} \quad \tau_2 = \frac{Tol}{||P_4 P_3||}. \tag{10}$$

If $\tau_1 \leq \lambda_1 \leq 1 - \tau_1$ and $\tau_2 \leq \lambda_2 \leq 1 - \tau_2$, two lines cross each other, if $(\tau_1 \leq \lambda_1 \leq 1 - \tau_1$ and $(|\lambda_2| < \tau_2$ or $|\lambda_2 - 1| < \tau_2))$ or $(\tau_2 \leq \lambda_2 \leq 1 - \tau_2$ and $(|\lambda_1| < \tau_1$ or $|\lambda_1 - 1| < \tau_1))$, two lines have a T-like intersection, and if $(|\lambda_1| < \tau_1$ or $|\lambda_1 - 1| < \tau_1)$ and $(|\lambda_2| < \tau_2$ or $|\lambda_2 - 1| < \tau_2)$, two lines intersect at the end-points within the given tolerance. Then, the intersection point $[r\ c]'$ can be found by substituting λ_1 into the Eq. (4) as

$$\begin{bmatrix} r \\ c \end{bmatrix} = \begin{bmatrix} r_1 \\ c_1 \end{bmatrix} + \lambda_1 \begin{bmatrix} r_2 - r_1 \\ c_2 - c_1 \end{bmatrix}. \tag{11}$$

Examples for the pre-processing steps are given in Figure 1.

2.2 Texture Histogram

The features for each pair of intersecting line segments consist of the angle between two lines and the ratio of mean gray level inside the region spanned by that angle to the mean gray level outside that region. Angle values are in the range $[0°, 180°]$. An example for region convention is given in Figure 2. Since the possible range of ratio values is infinite, we restrict them to the range $[0, 1)$ by taking the reciprocal if the inner region is brighter than the outer region.

The final features form a two-dimensional space of angles and the corresponding ratios, which is then partitioned into a fixed set of Q cells. The feature vector for each image is designed to be the Q-dimensional vector which has for its q'th component the number of angle-ratio pairs that fall into that q'th cell. As can be seen in Figure 3(a), these features do not have a uniform

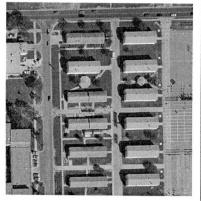

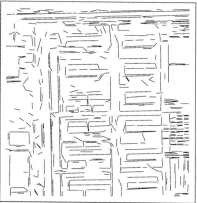

(a) Grayscale image.

(b) Extracted lines after line detection operator.

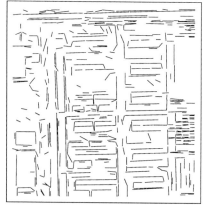

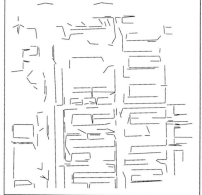

(c) Accepted lines after line selection operator.

(d) Resulting lines after line grouping operator.

Figure 1. Line selection and grouping pre-processing steps.

distribution so we use vector quantization [21] to form the Q-cell partition. Resulting partitions and their centroids for an example of 20 cells are given in Figure 3(b).

3 Variances of Gray Level Spatial Dependencies

Structural approaches to texture analysis use the idea that texture is composed of primitives with different properties appearing in particular spatial

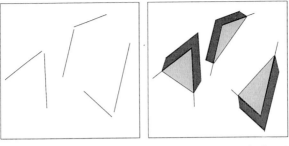

(a) Pairs of intersecting
lines.

(b) Regions used for
mean calculation.

Figure 2. Examples of region convention for mean ratio calculation. Light and dark shaded regions show the *in* and *out* regions respectively.

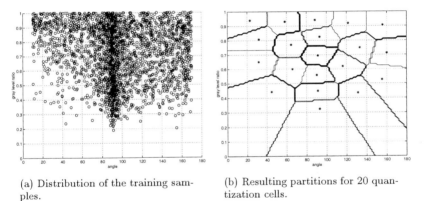

(a) Distribution of the training samples.

(b) Resulting partitions for 20 quantization cells.

Figure 3. Line-Angle-Ratio feature space distribution and centroids of the resulting partitions.

arrangements. On the other hand, statistical approaches try to model texture using statistical distributions either in the spatial domain or in a transform domain. One way to combine these two approaches is to define texture as being specified by the statistical distribution of the properties of different textural primitives occurring at different spatial relationships.

This information can be summarized in two-dimensional co-occurrence matrices that are matrices of relative frequencies $P(i, j; d, \theta)$ with which two pixels separated by distance d at orientation θ occur in the image, one with gray level i and the other with gray level j. These matrices are symmetric and can be normalized by dividing each entry in a matrix by the number of neighboring pixels used in computing that matrix.

The initial work on co-occurrence matrices [15] and some comparative studies [10,26] showed that gray level spatial dependency matrices were very successful in discriminating images with relatively homogeneous textures. Weszka *et al.* [31] discussed that if a texture is coarse and the distance d used to compute the co-occurrence matrix is small compared to the sizes of the texture elements, pairs of pixels at separation d should usually have similar gray levels. This means that high values in the matrix $P(i, j; d, \theta)$ should be concentrated on or near its main diagonal. Conversely, for a fine texture, if d is comparable to the texture element size, then the gray levels of points separated by d should often be quite different, so that values in $P(i, j; d, \theta)$ should be spread out relatively uniformly. Similarly, if a texture is directional, i.e. coarser in one direction than another, the degree of spread of the values about the main diagonal in $P(i, j; d, \theta)$ should vary with the orientation θ. Thus texture directionality can be analyzed by comparing spread measures of $P(i, j; d, \theta)$ for various orientations. Example co-occurrence matrices are given in Figure 4.

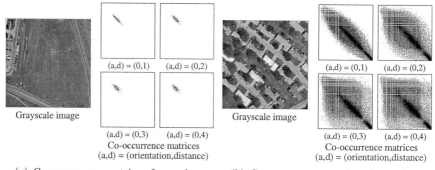

(a) Co-occurrence matrices for an image with a small amount of local spatial variations.

(b) Co-occurrence matrices for an image with a large amount of local spatial variations.

Figure 4. Example co-occurrence matrices.

3.1 Pre-processing

Before computing co-occurrence matrices we use equal probability quantization [15] to make the features invariant to distortions resulting in monotonic gray level transformations. We use 64 quantization levels (N_g) which performed the best among 16, 32 and 64 levels in terms of "total cost" that will be defined in Section 5. In the literature, usually a small number of levels were used because the images under consideration usually contained homogeneous textures, but our images are much more complex than those images and a small number of levels causes significant information loss.

3.2 Co-occurrence Variance

In order to use the information contained in the gray level co-occurrence matrices, Haralick *et al.* [15] defined 14 statistical measures. Since many distances and orientations result in a large amount of computation, we decided to use only the variance [3]

$$v(d, \theta) = \sum_{i=0}^{N_g-1} \sum_{j=0}^{N_g-1} (i - j)^2 P(i, j; d, \theta) \tag{12}$$

which is a difference moment of P and measures the contrast in the image. It will have a large value for images which have a large amount of local spatial variation in gray levels and a smaller value for images with spatially uniform gray level distributions. Gotlieb and Kreyszig [13] used heuristic selection methods to select the best subset of features for co-occurrence matrices and found out that the variance feature performed the best.

4 Multi-Scale Texture Analysis

Line-angle-ratio features capture the global spatial organization in an image by using relative orientations of lines extracted from it; therefore, they can be regarded as a macro-texture measure but are not effective if the image does not have any line content. On the other hand, co-occurrence variances capture local spatial variations of gray levels in the image; therefore, they are effective if the image is dominated by a fine, coarse, directional, or repetitive texture and can be regarded as a micro-texture measure. Another important difference is that line-angle-ratio features are invariant to rotation because they use relative orientations. On the contrary, co-occurrence variances are not rotation invariant because they are angularly dependent. If one also wants rotation invariance for these features, the feature vector can be modified by averaging the feature values for each distance over all orientations. [15]

In order to approximately equalize ranges of the features and make them have approximately the same effect in the computation of similarity, each component x in the feature vector is normalized as $y = F_x(x)$, where $F_x(\cdot)$ is the cumulative distribution function of that component. This makes y a random variable uniformly distributed in the $[0, 1]$ interval. Then, both feature vectors are appended to form the final vector. In the rest of the paper size of a feature vector will be denoted by Q.

5   Feature Selection

In a content-based retrieval system, features that are used to represent images should have close values for similar images and significantly different values for dissimilar ones. In many complex feature extraction algorithms, there are many parameters that, when varied, result in a large number of possible feature measurements. These high dimensional feature spaces may cause a problem of having less significant or even redundant features that contribute very little in the decision process.

Most of the times this feature selection process is done heuristically. Formal methods from the statistical pattern recognition literature include algorithms to form a new set of features from a set of available ones either by selecting a subset or by combining them into new features. [9,32,25,17] Only a few researchers [27,24,7] presented feature selection algorithms in their papers on database retrieval. Manjunath and Ma [24] used the total spectral energy to select among many possible Gabor filters and Carson et al. [7] used the minimum description length principle to select the number of Gaussians that best model the feature space.

We use a two-class pattern classification approach to find statistical measures of how well some of the features perform better than others. In doing so, we define two classes, the relevance class $\mathcal{A}$ and the irrelevance class $\mathcal{B}$, in order to classify image pairs as similar or dissimilar. Assume that we are given two sets of image pairs for the relevance and irrelevance classes respectively. [4,2] Differences of feature vectors for each image pair are assumed to have a normal distribution and sample means $\mu_{\mathcal{A}}$ and $\mu_{\mathcal{B}}$ and sample covariance matrices $\Sigma_{\mathcal{A}}$ and $\Sigma_{\mathcal{B}}$ are estimated using the training data. According to our experiments, the line-angle-ratio feature differences follow double-exponential distributions and the co-occurrence feature differences follow normal distributions. [5] Modeling the joint feature differences using a multivariate normal density worked better than using independently fitted double-exponentials or normals because of the covariance matrix that captures the correlation between features.

5.1   Classification Tests

Given a groundtruth image pair (n,m) with Q-dimensional feature vectors $x^{(n)}$ and $y^{(m)}$ respectively, first the difference $d = x^{(n)} - y^{(m)}$ is computed. From Bayes' law, the probability that these images are relevant is $P(\mathcal{A}|d) = P(d|\mathcal{A})P(\mathcal{A})/P(d)$ and that they are irrelevant is $P(\mathcal{B}|d) = P(d|\mathcal{B})P(\mathcal{B})/P(d)$.

The image pair is assigned to the relevance class if $P(\mathcal{A}|d) > P(\mathcal{B}|d)$, and to the irrelevance class otherwise. This can be written as

$$\text{Assign to } \mathcal{A} \text{ if } \frac{P(\mathcal{A}|d)}{P(\mathcal{B}|d)} > 1. \tag{13}$$

Assuming that both classes are equally likely, (13) becomes the likelihood ratio

$$\frac{P(d|\mathcal{A})}{P(d|\mathcal{B})} = \frac{P(d|\mu_{\mathcal{A}}, \Sigma_{\mathcal{A}})}{P(d|\mu_{\mathcal{B}}, \Sigma_{\mathcal{B}})}$$

$$= \frac{\frac{1}{(2\pi)^{Q/2}|\Sigma_{\mathcal{A}}|^{1/2}} e^{-(d-\mu_{\mathcal{A}})'\Sigma_{\mathcal{A}}^{-1}(d-\mu_{\mathcal{A}})/2}}{\frac{1}{(2\pi)^{Q/2}|\Sigma_{\mathcal{B}}|^{1/2}} e^{-(d-\mu_{\mathcal{B}})'\Sigma_{\mathcal{B}}^{-1}(d-\mu_{\mathcal{B}})/2}} \tag{14}$$

$$> 1.$$

After taking the natural logarithm of (14) and eliminating some constants, we obtain

$$(d-\mu_{\mathcal{A}})'\Sigma_{\mathcal{A}}^{-1}(d-\mu_{\mathcal{A}})/2 < (d-\mu_{\mathcal{B}})'\Sigma_{\mathcal{B}}^{-1}(d-\mu_{\mathcal{B}})/2 + \ln\frac{|\Sigma_{\mathcal{B}}|^{1/2}}{|\Sigma_{\mathcal{A}}|^{1/2}}. \tag{15}$$

Therefore, if the difference d of the feature vectors of two images satisfy the inequality in (15), this image pair is assigned to the relevance class, otherwise it is assigned to the irrelevance class.

5.2 Experimental Set-up

Suitable measures for the classification performance are misdetection and false alarm. In content-based retrieval we are more concerned with misdetection because we want to retrieve all the images similar to the query image. False alarm rate is also important because the purpose of querying a database is to retrieve similar images only, not all of them. We define total cost as 3 misdetection and 2 false alarm and use it as the criterion for "goodness", i.e. if a subset of features has a small total cost compared to others, it is called "good".

If the dimension of the feature space is large, it is computationally too expensive to do classification tests using all possible subsets of the features. In our work, first, we do tests using only one of the features at a time. The second test, which shrinks down feature sets, is done by first computing the total cost using all Q features. The feature with the worst total cost is discarded and the total cost using the remaining Q-1 features is computed. Then, the worst feature among the remaining Q-1 features is discarded and this procedure continues until one feature is left. A third test, which builds up feature sets, is done by starting with the total cost for each individual feature and selecting the best one. Given this best one, pairs of features are formed using one of the remaining features and this best feature. Total cost is computed for each pair and the one having the smallest cost is selected. Given the best two features, next, triplets of features are formed using one of the remaining features and these two best features. This procedure continues until all or a preselected number of features are used. These tests do not guarantee the optimal subset of features is found but they allow us to select a suboptimal subset without doing an exhaustive search.

6 Experiments and Results

6.1 Feature Selection

The images in our database come from the Fort Hood Data [1] of the RADIUS Project and also from the LANDSAT and Defense Meteorological Satellite Program (DMSP) Satellites. The RADIUS images consist of visible light aerial images of the Fort Hood area in Texas, USA. The LANDSAT images are from a remote sensing image collection. The test database for feature selection contains 10,410 256 × 256 images with a total of 38,240 groundtruth image pairs. Therefore, experiments for each parameter combination tested consist of classifying approximately 38,000 image pairs.

Line-Angle-Ratio Statistics:

The goal of these feature selection tests is to select the quantizer that performs the best. In order to reduce the search space, we consider only 15, 20 and 25 as the possible number of quantization cells. The quantizer with 15 cells resulted in a total cost of 30.20% whereas quantizers with 20 and 25 cells had 30.05% and 30.22% total costs respectively. As a result, we decided to use the quantizer with 20 cells.

Co-occurrence Variances:

The goal of our feature selection tests is to select the set of distances, among distances of 1 to 20 pixels, that perform the best according to the classification criteria. Each distance considered here is a combination of four features which correspond to variances computed at 0, 45, 90 and 135 degree orientations for that distance.

Results of the feature selection tests are given in Figure 5. In the experiments, building up feature sets decreased the total cost faster than shrinking down the set of all features. Another observation was that after using approximately 2 or 3 distances, total cost did not decrease much. As a result, using the distances 1 and 20 together had the minimum total cost of 29.36% among all the possible combinations of 2 distances. This resulted in an 8-dimensional feature vector.

When we consider the Remote Sensing Dataset and the Fort Hood Dataset separately, smaller distances resulted in smaller total costs for Remote Sensing images, while smaller total costs were obtained using large distances for Fort Hood images. This is consistent with the results of Weszka et al. [31] who stated that co-occurrence matrices computed for small distances performed better for a LANDSAT dataset. We believe that the reason for this is the strong micro-scale texture information in Remote Sensing images in contrast to larger structures in the Fort Hood images.

Although these feature selection tests do not guarantee to have an optimal solution, they resulted in a suboptimal one in 1,560 classification tests without using exhaustive search which would then require $2^{20} - 1$ classification tests.

6.2 Retrieval Performance

Two traditional measures for retrieval performance in the information retrieval literature are precision and recall. Precision is defined as the percentage of retrieved images that are actually relevant and recall is defined as the percentage of relevant images that are retrieved. For these tests, we randomly selected 340 images from the total of 10,410 and formed a groundtruth of 7 categories; parking lots, roads, residential areas, landscapes, LANDSAT USA, DMSP North Pole and LANDSAT Chernobyl. Likelihood values [2] which were derived from Eq. (15) were used to rank the database images. Average precision was used to evaluate the retrieval performance.

For comparison, UCSB's Gabor texture features, [24] IBM's QBIC texture features [12] and TUT's moments texture features [8] were also tested with Euclidean distance as the distance measure. Gabor features result in a 60-dimensional vector of means and variances of the image values filtered by a Gabor filter bank of 5 scales and 6 orientations. QBIC features result in a 4-dimensional vector of coarseness, contrast, directionality and orientation. Moments features result in a 36-dimensional vector of the means, variances, medians and absolute median deviations of the image values filtered by moment filters of up to 3rd order (which makes 9 2-dimensional filters).

Precision averaged over all 340 images when 12 images were retrieved was 0.73, 0.83, 0.48, and 0.51 for the ISL features, Gabor features, QBIC features, and moments features respectively. In most of the groundtruth groups, our features performed similarly to the Gabor features and both of them always performed significantly better than both QBIC and moments features. Figure 6 shows the average precision for some of the groundtruth

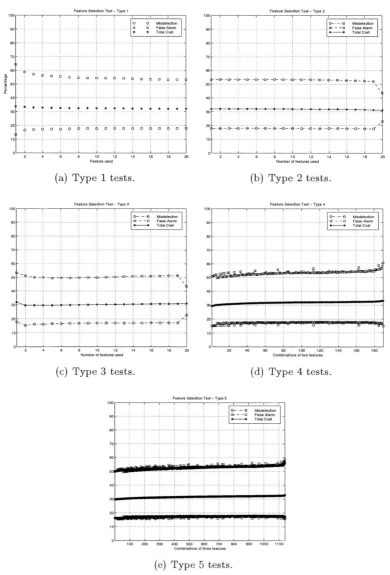

(a) Type 1 tests.

(b) Type 2 tests.

(c) Type 3 tests.

(d) Type 4 tests.

(e) Type 5 tests.

Figure 5. Feature selection tests for co-occurrence variances. Type 1 tests are done using only one feature at a time, type 2 tests are done using all features first and discarding the worst features one by one, type 3 tests are done using the best feature first and adding the next best features one by one, type 4 tests are done using all possible combinations of 2 features, type 5 tests are done using all possible combinations of 3 features. The criterion for "goodness" is the total cost which is plotted as (star,*).

groups. The feature extraction time for our features was approximately 30 times faster than that of the Gabor features. Some example queries are shown in Figure 7. More examples and our groundtruth data set can be found at http://isl.ee.washington.edu/~aksoy/research/database.shtml.

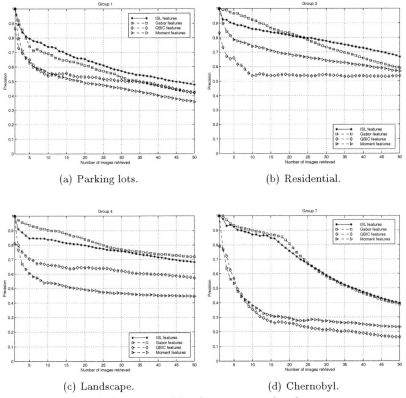

(a) Parking lots.

(b) Residential.

(c) Landscape.

(d) Chernobyl.

Figure 6. Average precision for some groundtruth groups.

Feature space visualizations for our features and the other features are given in Figure 8. Each feature is first normalized by a transformation to a Uniform[0,1] random variable using its marginal cumulative distribution function. Then, the high-dimensional feature space is projected into the first three principal components to reduce the dimensionality and Sammon's nonlinear mapping algorithm [18] is used to refine the projections. These plots show how the feature space is structured compared to the manually generated groundtruth. Although there is no perfect mapping to 3D, it can be seen

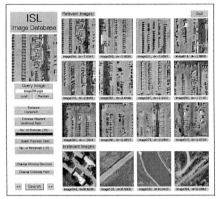

(a) Example query for parking lots.

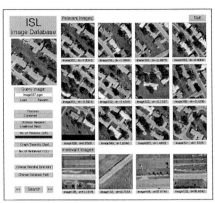

(b) Example query for residential.

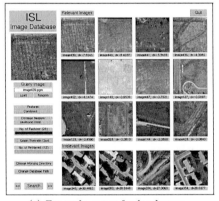

(c) Example query for landscape.

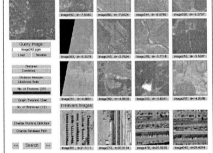

(d) Example query for Chernobyl.

Figure 7. Retrieval examples with the upper left image as the query. Among the retrieved images, first three rows show the 12 most relevant images in descending order of similarity and the last row shows the 4 most irrelevant images in descending order of dissimilarity.

from Figure 8 that our features and Gabor features create a feature space structure that is closer to the manual groundtruth. Some of the individual query results look much better than the average precision results for some groundtruth groups. The reason for this are the difficulties encountered during assigning complex aerial images (e.g. roads and buildings) into single categories. Another observation is that different features can represent different classes of images well so the retrieval performance can be improved significantly if we can find effective ways of combining features from multiple feature extraction algorithms.

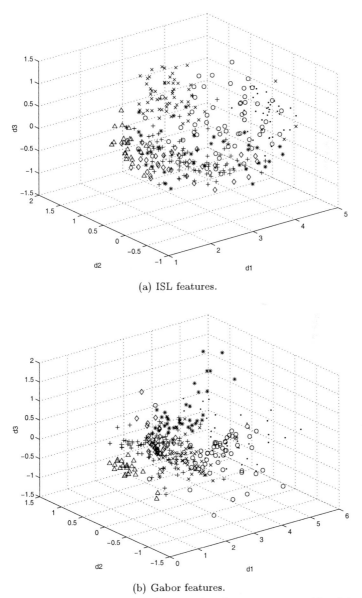

(a) ISL features.

(b) Gabor features.

Figure 8. Feature space projections. The groundtruth groups are: parking lots (point), roads (circle), residential areas (x-mark), landscapes (plus), LANDSAT USA (star), DMSP North Pole (diamond) and LANDSAT Chernobyl (triangle).

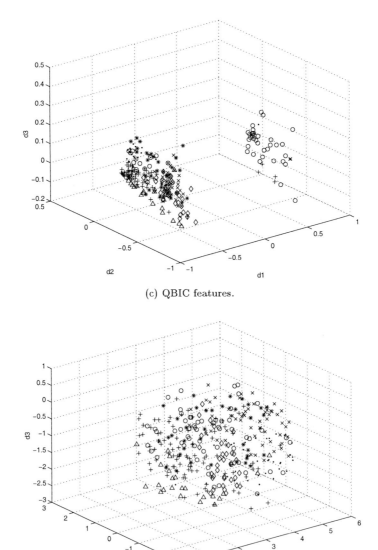

(c) QBIC features.

(d) Moments features.

Figure 8. Feature space projections (cont.).

7 Conclusions

We described easy-to-compute but effective low-level textural features. The first set of features capture the global spatial organization in the image using the edge and line information. The second set of features are effective if the image is dominated by a fine, coarse, directional, or repetitive texture. Some key aspects of this work include a statistical line selection algorithm that uses hypothesis testing to eliminate lines that do not have significant difference between the gray level distributions in the regions on their right and left, and also feature selection tests to determine the parameters of the feature extraction algorithms to avoid having less significant or even redundant features that increase computation but contribute very little in the decision process.

Precision averaged over 340 randomly selected queries on a database of approximately 10,000 images was used to evaluate the retrieval performance in comparative tests with three other texture analysis algorithms. These tests showed that our features had an average precision of 0.73 when 12 images were retrieved and performed significantly better than two of the other features while having similar performance as the third one. They can be combined with other features to further improve the performance and make better inferences about the high-level descriptions of the images.

Acknowledgments

The authors would like to thank Tom Minka from MIT Media Laboratory, USA, for the code for QBIC texture features, Bogdan Cramariuc from Tampere University of Technology, Finland, for the code for moment texture features, and Wei-Ying Ma from the University of California, Santa Barbara, USA, for the code for Gabor texture features.

References

1. *Fort Hood Datasets*, http://www.mbvlab.wpafb.af.mil/public/sdms/datasets/fthood/index.htm.
2. S. Aksoy, *Textural features for content-based image database retrieval*, Master's thesis, University of Washington, Seattle, WA, June 1998, Online: http://isl.ee.washington.edu/~aksoy/thesis.shtml.
3. S. Aksoy and R. M. Haralick, *Content-based image database retrieval using variances of gray level spatial dependencies*, Proceedings of IAPR International Workshop on Multimedia Information Analysis and Retrieval (Hong Kong), August 13–14 1998, as Lecture Notes in Computer Science,

vol. 1464, pp. 3–19.

4. ———, *Textural features for image database retrieval*, Proceedings of IEEE Workshop on Content-Based Access of Image and Video Libraries, CVPR'98 (Santa Barbara, CA), June 1998, pp. 45–49.

5. ———, *Probabilistic vs. geometric similarity measures for image retrieval*, Proceedings of IEEE Conference on Computer Vision and Pattern Recognition (Hilton Head Island, South Carolina), June 2000.

6. J. Canny, *A computational approach to edge detection*, IEEE Transactions on Pattern Analysis and Machine Intelligence **8** (1986), 679–698.

7. C. Carson, S. Belongie, H. Greenspan, and J. Malik, *Region-based image querying*, Proceedings of IEEE Workshop on Content-Based Access of Image and Video Libraries, 1997.

8. F. A. Cheikh et al., *Muvis: A system for content-based indexing and retrieval in large image databases*, SPIE Storage and Retrieval of Image and Video Databases VII (San Jose, CA), January 1999, pp. 98–106.

9. Y. T. Chien, *A sequential decision model for selecting feature subsets in pattern recognition*, IEEE Transactions on Computers **C-20** (1971), no. 3, 282–290.

10. R. W. Conners and C. A. Harlow, *A theoretical comparison of texture algorithms*, IEEE Transactions on Pattern Analysis and Machine Intelligence **2** (1980), no. 3, 25–39.

11. A. Etemadi, *Robust segmentation of edge data*, IEE Image Processing Conference, 1992.

12. M. Flickner et al., *The QBIC project: Querying images by content using color, texture and shape*, SPIE Storage and Retrieval of Image and Video Databases, 1993, pp. 173–181.

13. C. C. Gotlieb and H. E. Kreyszig, *Texture descriptors based on co-occurrence matrices*, Computer Vision, Graphics, and Image Processing **51** (1990), no. 1, 70–86.

14. R. M. Haralick, *Statistical and structural approaches to texture*, Proceedings of the IEEE **67** (1979), no. 5, 786–804.

15. R. M. Haralick, K. Shanmugam, and I. Dinstein, *Textural features for image classification*, IEEE Transactions on Systems, Man, and Cybernetics **SMC-3** (1973), no. 6, 610–621.

16. R. M. Haralick and L. G. Shapiro, *Glossary of computer vision terms*, Pattern Recognition **24** (1991), no. 1, 69–93.

17. A. K. Jain and R. Dubes, *Feature definition in pattern recognition with small sample size*, Pattern Recognition **10** (1978), no. 2, 85–97.

18. J. W. Sammon Jr., *A nonlinear mapping for data structure analysis*, IEEE Transactions on Computers **C-18** (1969), no. 5, 401–409.

19. P. M. Kelly and T. M. Cannon, *CANDID: Comparison algorithm for navigating digital image databases*, Proceedings of the Seventh International Working Conference on Scientific and Statistical Database Management, September 1994, pp. 252–258.

20. C. S. Li and V. Castelli, *Deriving texture set for content based retrieval of satellite image database*, IEEE International Conference on Image Processing, 1997, pp. 576–579.

21. Y. Linde, A. Buzo, and R. M. Gray, *An algorithm for vector quantizer design*, IEEE Transactions on Communications **COM-28** (1980), 84–95.

22. F. Liu and R. W. Picard, *Periodicity, directionality, and randomness: Wold features for image modeling and retrieval*, IEEE Transactions on Pattern Analysis and Machine Intelligence **18** (1996), no. 7, 722–733.

23. W. Y. Ma and B. S. Manjunath, *NETRA: A toolbox for navigating large image databases*, Proceedings of IEEE International Conference on Image Processing, 1997.

24. B. S. Manjunath and W. Y. Ma, *Texture features for browsing and retrieval of image data*, IEEE Transactions on Pattern Analysis and Machine Intelligence **18** (1996), no. 8, 837–842.

25. P. M. Narendra and K. Fukunage, *A branch and bound algorithm for feature subset selection*, IEEE Transactions on Computers **C-26** (1977), no. 9, 917–922.

26. P. P. Ohanian and R. C. Dubes, *Performance evaluation for four classes of textural features*, Pattern Recognition **25** (1992), no. 8, 819–833.

27. A. Pentland, R. W. Picard, and S. Sclaroff, *Photobook: Content-based manipulation of image databases*, SPIE Storage and Retrieval of Image and Video Databases II, February 1994, pp. 34–47.

28. J. R. Smith, *Integrated spatial and feature image systems: Retrieval, analysis and compression*, Ph.D. thesis, Columbia University, 1997.

29. H. Tamura, S. Mori, and T. Yamawaki, *Textural features corresponding to visual perception*, IEEE Transactions on Systems, Man, and Cybernetics **SMC-8** (1978), no. 6, 460–473.

30. M. Tuceryan and A. K. Jain, Handbook of Pattern Recognition and Computer Vision, ch. Texture Analysis, pp. 235–276, World Scientific Publishing Company, River Edge, NJ, 1993, pp. 235–276.

31. J. S. Weszka, C. R. Dyer, and A. Rosenfeld, *A comparative study of texture measures for terrain classification*, IEEE Transactions on Systems, Man, and Cybernetics **SMC-6** (1976), no. 4, 269–285.

32. A. Whitney, *A direct method of nonparametric measurement selection*, IEEE Transactions on Computers **20** (1971), no. 9, 1100–1103.

SCALE AND ORIENTATION-INVARIANT TEXTURE MATCHING FOR IMAGE RETRIEVAL

WEE KHENG LEOW

School of Computing, National University of Singapore, Lower Kent Ridge Road,
Singapore 119260
E-mail: leowwk@comp.nus.edu.sg

SEOW YONG LAI

DSO National Laboratories, 20 Science Park Drive, Singapore 118230
E-mail: lseowyon@dso.org.sg

Texture-based image retrieval is a very difficult task, especially for retrieving images of natural scene. Such images contain multiple texture patterns that may vary in intensity, scale, and orientation but still look the same to humans. Existing methods have been successful in retrieving images that contain single uniform texture but their performance often deteriorate when retrieving natural scene images. This article presents an invariant texture matching method that can retrieve images containing texture patterns that differ in intensity, scale, and orientation from the query texture. Experimental results show that the invariant method performs better than existing methods especially in retrieving natural scene images.

1 Introduction

Retrieval of images, especially images of natural scene, based on texture is a very difficult task. Such images contain a wide variety of natural texture such as bricks, wire mesh, sand, and grass patches. Non-uniform lighting conditions resulting from shadows, time of the day, etc. can alter the apparent brightness of the texture. In addition, texture patterns in natural scene images tend to vary smoothly in scale and orientation due to perspective distortion. Nevertheless, humans still perceive them as the same texture. Therefore, texture matching should be invariant to texture intensity, scale, and orientation.

Main texture classification techniques used for content-based image retrieval can be categorized into two approaches: statistical and spectral. Statistical methods characterize texture in terms of local statistical measures (e.g., coarseness, directionality, and contrast) [1], simultaneous autoregressive models (SAR) [2], or Markov random field models [3]. Variations of these methods have been shown to be rotation and scale-invariant in classifying Brodatz textures [4,5]. In general, these models are good at modeling random patterns such as sand and pebbles but not so suitable for modeling highly structured patterns such as roof tiles and bricks. Liu and Picard [6] showed that the

SAR method does not return satisfying results in retrieving images of structured patterns. Among these methods, Tamura's texture features [1] are used in IBM's QBIC [7] and Markov random field model is used in MIT's Photo-Book [6]. In addition, MIT's PhotoBook also uses Discrete Fourier Transform to extract texture features.

The spectral approach is based on the response of a set of band-pass filters, usually the 2D Gabor filters [8]. Each filter responds most strongly to a selected spatial-frequency and orientation bands. The advantage of this approach is that both scale and orientation information about the texture can be captured by the filters. This method has been used extensively for classifying plane textures such as Brodatz textures and aerial images [8,9,10,11]. It has also been adopted in the NeTra image retrieval system [12].

Existing texture matching methods, for example [1,6,7,12], can effectively handle images containing single texture patterns that are uniform in scale and orientation. However, their performance often deteriorate when they are used to match texture patterns that differ in scale and orientation. This article presents a texture matching method that is invariant to intensity, scale, and orientation of texture. Experimental results show that it performs better than existing methods especially in retrieving images of natural scenes.

2 Texture Feature Extraction

To perform texture matching, texture features are first extracted from the images, and the images are segmented into regions each containing a homogeneous texture pattern. Texture features are extracted from an image using a set of Gabor filters [8]:

$$h(x,y) = \frac{1}{2\pi\lambda\sigma^2} \exp\left[-\frac{(x'/\lambda)^2 + y'^2}{2\sigma^2}\right] \exp(2\pi j f x') \qquad (1)$$

where $(x', y') = (x\cos\theta + y\sin\theta, -x\sin\theta + y\cos\theta)$ are rotated coordinates oriented at angle θ from the x-axis, λ is the aspect ratio, and σ is the scale parameter. The maximum spatial frequency is set at 0.3 cycle per pixel because Gabor filters with spatial-frequency higher than 0.3 cycle per pixel cannot be accurately represented in digital form [8]. The spatial frequency bandwidth is set at 0.5 octave so that 6 frequency channels can cover the spatial frequency range of most texture patterns. The orientation bandwidth is set at 45°, which allows 8 orientation channels to cover all possible orientations. Hence, a total of 48 filters with 6 spatial frequencies and 8 orientations are used.

An input image $I(x,y)$ is filtered by a set of Gabor filters with different frequencies f and orientations θ:

$$\begin{aligned}
e_{c,f\theta}(x,y) &= I(x,y) * h_{c,f\theta}(x,y) \\
e_{s,f\theta}(x,y) &= I(x,y) * h_{s,f\theta}(x,y)
\end{aligned} \tag{2}$$

where $h_{c,f\theta}(x,y)$ and $h_{s,f\theta}(x,y)$ are the real and imaginary components of the Gabor function. The Gabor channels' output energy is computed as:

$$E_{f\theta}(x,y) = e_{c,f\theta}^2(x,y) + e_{s,f\theta}^2(x,y) \ . \tag{3}$$

After Gabor filtering, the channels' outputs are smoothed by Gaussian filters to remove local variations introduced by the sinusoidal terms in the Gabor functions. The channels' outputs at each pixel location are further normalized to remove intensity variation by dividing the energy value of each channel by the largest value at that location:

$$G_{f\theta}(x,y) = \frac{E_{f\theta}(x,y)}{\max\limits_{f,\theta} E_{f\theta}(x,y)} \ . \tag{4}$$

Since the energy of Gabor output is proportional to the (square of the) image intensity, the normalization process will remove variations in Gabor outputs due to differences in texture image intensity. The normalized Gabor outputs now form a multi-dimensional texture feature vector at each pixel location that is invariant to image intensity.

Once the feature vectors are extracted, a region segmentation algorithm is applied to segment the image into regions each containing a homogeneous texture. For the purpose of image retrieval, the region segmentation algorithm need not localize the region boundaries precisely. It only has to ensure that each region contains a single texture pattern. In the current implementation, segmentation is performed by computing the normalized vector dot product of the texture features at neighboring positions, and grouping positions with large product into the same region.

3 Invariant Texture Matching Method

The invariant texture matching method consists of two steps: (1) feature transformation and (2) feature matching. The first step transforms the texture feature vectors into a texture space that is invariant to scale and orientation. The second step performs matching both in the invariant texture space as well as using the original feature vectors.

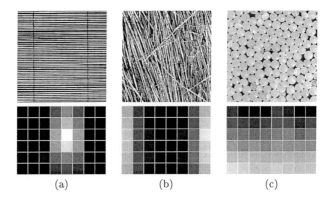

(a) (b) (c)

Figure 1. The structures of different textures (top row) manifest as different patterns in the 2D representations of Gabor feature vectors (bottom row). In the 2D representations, spatial frequency increases from bottom up along the vertical axis, and orientation changes from left to right along the horizontal axis and wraps around. Each square represents the output of a Gabor channel, with light squares denoting large outputs.

3.1 Feature Transformation

Texture feature transformation is performed based on an important characteristic of the Gabor feature vectors, which can be represented in a 2-dimensional pattern with frequency increasing along the vertical axis and orientation along the horizontal axis (Fig. 1). Three distinct patterns are observed for three extreme types of textures. Highly structured texture with specific scale and orientation has localized peaks in the 2D representation (Fig. 1a). Oriented texture with a specific orientation and a range of scales has a column-shaped pattern in the 2D representation (Fig. 1b). Granular texture with a specific scale and a range of orientations has a row-shaped pattern (Fig. 1c). These distinct patterns correspond to three important texture characteristics: structuredness, orientedness, and granularity. They form three axes of the invariant texture space. A typical texture would contain a mixture of these three texture characteristics. Different texture patterns would have different 2D representations and would map into different points in the texture space. This method of representing various textures is known as *distributed representation* in the Neural Networks literature [13].

Interestingly, the texture categories defined above correspond closely to the texture characteristics used in the Wold texture model. However, the texture spaces defined in the two models are not identical. In particular, the Wold model defines periodicity, directionality, and randomness as the texture dimensions. The invariant texture space, on the other hand, defines structuredness (similar to periodicity), orientedness (similar to directionality), and granularity as the texture dimensions. Randomness of the Wold model corresponds to a region in the invariant space rather than a dimension.

Similar texture categories have been found to be important texture attributes in the study of Rao and Lohse on human's perception of texture similarity [14]. In the study, repetitiveness, directionality and complexity are the three texture attributes found to be most important to human's perception of texture and they correspond to the structuredness, orientedness and randomness of the invariant texture space.

We have proved mathematically for a sinusoidal texture that a change of its spatial frequency or orientation does not alter its corresponding 2D Gabor pattern but only shifts the pattern along the vertical or horizontal axis [15]. Empirical results show that this property is largely preserved for real images of natural textures (e.g., Fig. 2).

The amounts of texture characteristics possessed by a texture are computed using a template matching method. Three distinct masks are devised to detect the presence of local peaks, columns of peaks, and rows of peaks in the 2D representation:

$$c_i = \max_{f\theta}(\mathbf{G}_{f\theta} \star \mathbf{T}_i) \tag{5}$$

where c_i is the amount of texture characteristic of type i for $i = 1, 2, 3$, $\mathbf{G}_{f\theta}$ is a 2D representation of Gabor texture feature, $\mathbf{T}_i$ is the mask, and $\star$ denotes the normalized cross-correlation operation. The mask values are obtained using a training method similar to the "tuned" masks method [4].

Since a scale or orientation change in a texture results in only a shift of its 2D Gabor representation along the vertical or horizontal axis, roughly the same amounts of texture characteristics are contained in the 2D Gabor representations of the scaled and rotated versions of a texture. The template matching operation (Eq. 5) will detect the amounts of texture characteristics present in a texture regardless of the locations (i.e., spatial frequencies and orientations) of the characteristics patterns (Fig. 1) in the 2D Gabor representation. Therefore, it transforms the texture feature vectors, which contain frequency and orientation information, into vector points in the 3D texture space which is invariant to scale and orientation. Together with normalization of texture energy (Eq. 4), the vector points now correspond to intensity-, scale-, and orientation-invariant representations of the textures.

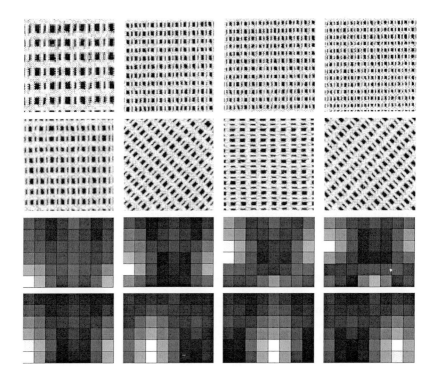

Figure 2. Feature pattern shifts according to changes in texture frequency and orientation. Top two rows show a simple texture in various scales and orientations. Last two rows show the feature patterns in the 2D representation, with frequency increasing from bottom up and orientation changing from left to right. As the frequency and orientation change, the feature pattern shifts along the vertical and horizontal axes.

3.2 Feature Matching

After feature transformation, the texture patterns can now be matched in the invariant texture space using simple Euclidean distance measure. The smaller the Euclidean distance between two vector points, the more similar are the corresponding texture patterns.

Ideally, texture patterns that differ only in scales and orientations should map to a single point in the texture space. In practice, however, due to limited resolution and the presence of image noise, these patterns actually map into a region in the texture space, and neighboring regions corresponding to similar looking textures may overlap. Consequently, ranking based on the Euclidean distance in the texture space alone may not accurately reflect the similarity between the texture patterns.

To improve the ranking of the textures, a rank refinement process is performed as follows. A texture t's original Gabor feature vector (Eq. 4) is compared with those of its nearest N neighbors down the ranked list. The comparison is performed using normalized vector dot product. Neighbors that are more similar to texture t are moved up the list whereas those that are less similar are moved down. This procedure is repeated for every texture in the ranked list.

After rank refinement, the ranked list of texture patterns is mapped into a ranked list of images by identifying the images that contain the texture patterns. An image may appear more than once in the ranked list if it contains multiple texture regions that match the query texture. The image instance that is at the top of the list is retained whereas the others are discarded. The final ranked list of images is the result of the invariant texture matching method.

4   Experimental Results

Extensive experiments have been conducted to compare the performance of the invariant texture matching method and existing methods. Two existing methods were considered:

1. matching method based on the texture model of Tamura et al. [1] because it is used in many existing image retrieval systems [7], and

2. matching method based on the Wold model because it has been reported to outperform other existing methods for retrieving Brodatz texture images [6]. It would be reasonable to regard the Wold method as a representative of the state-of-the-art texture-based image retrieval method.

The source codes of these methods were downloaded from the FTP sites vismod.www.media.mit.edu/pub/fliu/wold and /pub/tpminka/MRSAR.

The three texture matching methods were tested on retrieving both Brodatz textures and natural scene images. For Brodatz texture retrieval tests, each image in the Brodatz album provides nine 256×256 patches. A total of 1008 patches were cropped from the 112 images in the album. Texture patches that are perceptually identical are classified into the same group based on the work done by Ma and Manjunath [16]. A total of 38 texture groups were formed each containing 1 to 7 types of texture.

In a retrieval test, one of the texture patches served as the query texture and the three texture matching methods were executed to rank the other 1007

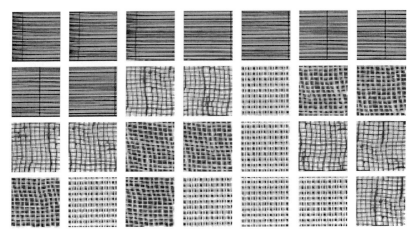

Figure 3. Sample Brodatz image patches retrieved using Tamura et al.'s texture features in decreasing order of similarity. The first patch is the query texture.

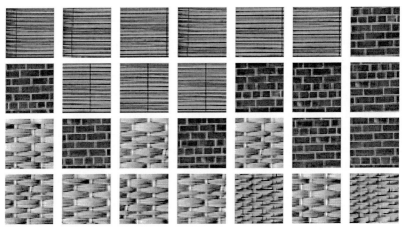

Figure 4. Sample Brodatz image patches retrieved using the Wold texture features in decreasing order of similarity. The first patch is the query texture.

patches. Sample retrieval results are shown in Figs. 3–5. The results show that the methods based on the Tamura features and the Wold model can retrieve texture patches that appear to be quite different from the query texture. On the other hand, the texture patches retrieved by the invariant matching method are more perceptually similar to the query texture, even when their

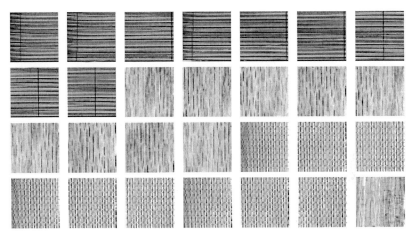

Figure 5. Sample Brodatz image patches retrieved by the invariant texture matching method in decreasing order of similarity. The first patch is the query texture.

Table 1. Performance of texture matching methods in retrieving Brodatz texture images. P_n and R_n are the normalized precision and recall rates, and diff is the improvement of the invariant method over the other methods.

query	Tamura		Wold		Invariant	
	P_n	R_n	P_n	R_n	P_n	R_n
D15	1.00	1.00	1.00	1.00	0.98	1.00
D31	0.65	0.85	0.70	0.81	0.58	0.75
D40	0.47	0.81	0.58	0.81	0.67	0.85
D49	1.00	1.00	0.99	1.00	1.00	1.00
D53	0.62	0.82	0.55	0.78	0.95	0.99
D66	0.43	0.61	0.85	0.96	0.62	0.86
D82	0.51	0.70	0.89	0.97	0.76	0.94
D96	0.70	0.87	0.72	0.93	0.84	0.94
D100	0.83	0.98	0.84	0.99	0.96	0.99
D112	0.87	0.97	0.92	0.98	0.83	0.97
mean	0.71	0.86	0.80	0.92	0.82	0.93
diff (%)	15.7	7.9	1.9	0.7	–	–

orientations differ from that of the query texture. Ten retrievals were performed using representatives of structured, oriented, granular, and random texture patterns as the query texture. Table 1 summarizes the performance of the three methods measured in terms of normalized precision and recall. The Wold method, with very high precision and recall, is indeed a very good

Table 2. Performance of the texture matching methods in retrieving natural scene images. P_n and R_n are the normalized precision and recall rates, and diff is the improvement of the invariant method over the other methods.

query	Tamura		Wold		Invariant	
	P_n	R_n	P_n	R_n	P_n	R_n
1	0.62	0.81	0.18	0.36	0.82	0.89
2	0.32	0.50	0.17	0.33	0.55	0.62
3	0.57	0.68	0.30	0.48	0.64	0.72
4	0.32	0.61	0.38	0.52	0.59	0.62
5	0.33	0.70	0.33	0.67	0.72	0.86
6	0.33	0.70	0.39	0.70	0.82	0.94
7	0.50	0.71	0.23	0.50	0.77	0.86
8	0.58	0.72	0.45	0.67	0.62	0.73
9	0.16	0.38	0.42	0.69	0.63	0.69
10	0.31	0.60	0.16	0.42	0.55	0.70
mean	0.40	0.64	0.30	0.53	0.67	0.76
diff (%)	66.1	19.0	122.9	42.9	–	–

method for retrieving Brodatz images [6]. Nevertheless, the invariant method can still perform slightly better than the Wold method.

In the natural image retrieval tests, 539 texture regions were extracted from 100 images of natural scene. In each retrieval, one of these texture patterns or a Brodatz texture patch was used as the query texture and the three texture matching methods were executed to rank the natural scene images. A sample retrieval result is shown in Fig. 6.

Ten retrievals were performed using representatives of structured, oriented, granular, and random texture patterns as the query texture. Table 2 summarizes the performance of the three methods in retrieving natural scene images. Surprisingly, the Wold method did not perform as well as the Tamura method in retrieving natural scene images. A possible explanation is that the Wold model uses Discrete Fourier Transform (DFT) to extract texture features. Unfortunately, DFT can be drastically affected by image inhomogeneity [6] such as scale and orientation variations due to perspective distortion. In contrast, the invariant method performs significantly better than the other two methods precisely because it is designed to handle variations in texture scale and orientation.

161

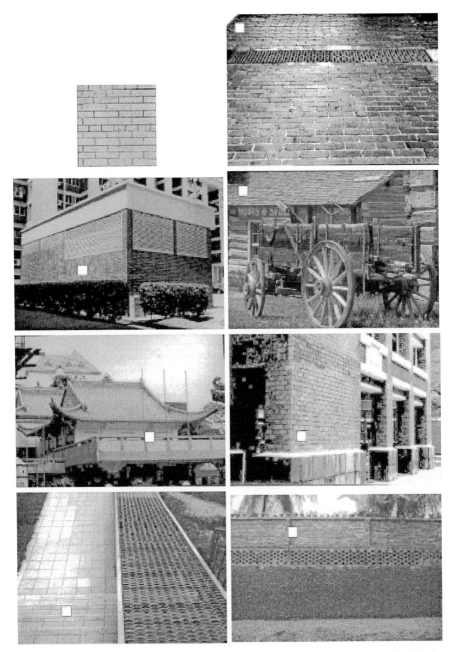

Figure 6. Sample natural scene images retrieved by the invariant matching method in decreasing order of similarity. The first image is the query texture. The white boxes in the images denote the regions that best match the query texture.

5 Conclusion

Texture matching for content-based image retrieval is a very difficult task, especially for retrieving natural scene images. These images can contain multiple texture patterns that vary in intensity due to different lighting conditions, and differ in scale and orientation due to perspective distortion. This article presented a texture matching method that is invariant to texture intensity, scale, and orientation. It extracts texture feature vectors using Gabor filters, transforms the feature vectors into an intensity-, scale-, and orientation-invariant texture space, compares texture similarity in the texture space, and refines texture ranking using the original Gabor feature vectors. Experimental results show that the invariant texture matching method outperforms existing methods in retrieving both Brodatz images and, especially, natural scene images.

Acknowledgement

This research is supported by NUS research grant RP950656.

References

1. H. Tamura, S. Mori, and T. Yamawaki. Textural features corresponding to visual perception. *IEEE Trans. on SMC*, 8(6):460–473, 1978.
2. J.C. Mao and A.K. Jain. Texture classification and segmentation using multiresolution simultaneous autoregressive models. *Pattern Recognition*, 25:173–188, 1992.
3. G.R. Cross and A.K. Jain. Markov random field texture models. *IEEE Trans. on PAMI*, 5:25–39, 1983.
4. J. You and H. A. Cohen. Classification and segmentation of rotated and scaled textured images using texture "tuned" masks. *Pattern Recognition*, 26(2):245–258, 1993.
5. F. S. Cohen, Z. Fan, and M. A. Patel. Classification of rotated and scaled textured images using Gaussian Markov random field models. *IEEE Trans. on PAMI*, 13(2):192–202, 1991.
6. F. Liu and R.W. Picard. Periodicity, directionality, and randomness: Wold features for image modeling and retrieval. *IEEE Trans. on PAMI*, 18(7):722–733, July, 1996.
7. J. Ashley, R. Barber, M. Flickner, J.L. Hafner, D. Lee, W. Niblack, and D. Petkovic. Automatic and semiautomatic methods for image annotation and retrieval in QBIC. In *Proceedings of SPIE Storage and Retrieval*

for Image and Video Databases III, pages 24–35, Feb 1995.

8. A.C. Bovik, M. Clark, and W.S. Geisler. Multichannel texture analysis using localized spatial filters. *IEEE Trans. on PAMI*, 12(1):55–73, 1990.

9. J. Bigün and J. M. H. Du Buf. *N*-folded symmetries by complex moments in Gabor space and their application to unsupervised texture segmentation. *IEEE Trans. on PAMI*, 16(1):80–87, 1994.

10. D. Dunn, W. E. Higgins, and J. Wakeley. Texture segmentation using 2-D Gabor elementary functions. *IEEE Trans. on PAMI*, 16(2):130–149, 1994.

11. A. K. Jain and F. Farrokhnia. Unsupervised texture segmentation using Gabor filters. *Pattern Recognition*, 24(12):1167–1186, 1991.

12. W.Y. Ma and B.S. Manjunath. NeTra: A toolbox for navigating large image databases. In *IEEE Conference on Image Processing*, volume 1, pages 568–571, Oct 1997.

13. G.E. Hinton, J.L. McClelland, and D.E. Rumelhart. Distributed representation. In D.E. Rumelhart and J.L. McClelland, editors, *Parallel Distributed Processing*. MIT Press, Cambridge, Massachusetts, 1986.

14. A.R. Rao and G.L. Lohse. Towards a texture naming system: Identifying relevant dimensions of texture. *IEEE Conference on Visualization*, pages 220–227, Oct 1993.

15. N. Zhang. Invariant texture segmentation for images of natural scene. Master's thesis, Dept. of Information Systems and Computer Science, National University of Singapore, 1997.

16. W.Y. Ma and B.S. Manjunath. Texture features and learning similarity. In *Proc. of IEEE CVPR*, pages 1160–1169, June, 1996.

A SURVEY OF TEXTURE-BASED METHODS FOR DOCUMENT LAYOUT ANALYSIS

OLEG OKUN[1,2] AND MATTI PIETIKÄINEN[1]

[1] *Department of Electrical Engineering, University of Oulu,*
P.O.Box 4500, FIN-90401 Oulu, FINLAND
E-mail:{mkp,oleg}@ee.oulu.fi

[2] *Institute of Engineering Cybernetics, National Academy of Sciences of Belarus,*
Surganov street 6, 220012 Minsk, BELARUS
E-mail:ogo@newman.basnet.minsk.by

Document layout analysis plays an important role in document image processing and recognition. Its purpose is to divide a document image into a number of regions, each of which contains homogeneous data of a particular class such as text, graphics or pictures. This operation is necessary because the data of each class will be further processed by different techniques. The layout analysis problem is often considered as texture segmentation and classification in the literature. In this paper, we review progress achieved in this area to date.

1 Introduction

Ordinary documents are paper-based media containing different classes of information such as text, graphics, and pictures. Document images, obtained through document digitisation with special input devices often called scanners, are electronic copies or analogues of the corresponding paper documents. However, these images, as they are, are not very useful and they occupy much memory space. That is, some kind of processing should be done before they are more suitable for data transmission, storage, or editing. One of the first tasks to be taken on is document layout analysis.

Document layout analysis deals with segmentation of a document image into homogeneous zones or regions and their classification. Each zone contains data belonging to one particular class. The classification can be done either during segmentation or after. In this paper, we assume that there are only four classes: text, background, binary graphics (line-arts, line-drawings), and greyscale pictures. These are the main classes of document images and they are analysed in many papers.

The methods developed for layout analysis can be divided into two classes: texture-based and non-texture-based. The texture-based methods consider a document image as a composite of textures of different classes. With this approach, various well-known texture segmentation and classification techniques can be used directly or with minor modifications. The non-texture-based methods apply other image processing techniques (for example, connected component analysis or various splitting-and-merging strategies) to this task and do not treat the image as texture. In this paper, we analyse existing texture-based methods and briefly compare them to the non-texture-based ones.

2   A survey of texture-based methods

When a document image is considered as texture, the text areas are assumed to have different texture features from the non-text ones. The text regions are modelled as regular periodic textures, because they contain text lines with the same orientation, and their intercharacter and interline spacings are approximately the same. In contrast to these, the non-text regions correspond to irregular textures. Therefore, the problem is how to separate two (or more) different texture classes. Examples of different textures in document images are shown in Fig. 1.

anisotropic therm
perties of CC tiles.
tile in the tube a
in that in the othe
eratures in the ar
1150°C and 35(

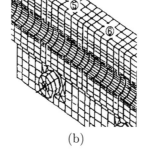

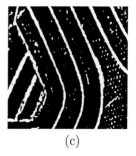

(a)   (b)   (c)

Figure 1. Different document zones can be associated with different texture classes. Text zones (a) can be viewed as a regular texture, while non-text zones (b) and (c) can be considered as irregular textures.

Our review is organised as follows. First we briefly introduce each method. Its initial conditions are considered in the heading "INPUT". Among these are the image resolution used and image type (binary or greyscale). The heading "ALGORITHM" describes the implementation of each method step by step. The parameters needed to be predefined are discussed in the heading "PARAMETERS". The output of the algorithm and the processing time are presented in the headings "OUTPUT" and "PROCESSING TIME", respectively. The good and weak points of each method are presented in the headings "ADVANTAGES" and "DISADVANTAGES".

2.1 The layout-driven technique

This method [12] was one of the first techniques using texture-based document image analysis. It relies on the rectangularity of page blocks and their separability from each other by sufficiently wide horizontal/vertical white spaces. The method was especially designed for documents of such a layout. The RLSA (run length smoothing algorithm) and RXYC (recursive X-Y cuts) methods are first applied to segment the document image into a number of homogeneous rectangular blocks that are further classified by using simple texture statistics based on the occurrence of the black and white run lengths within each region.

INPUT: Binary image of 100 or 200 dpi.

ALGORITHM:

Step 1. Page segmentation into rectangular blocks.

Step 2. Computation of matrices of texture statistics.

Step 3. Extraction of texture features from matrices.

Step 4. Block classification based on these features.

The first step employs RLSA and RXYC methods to segment the image into rectangular blocks containing homogeneous information.

Two matrices, called the black-white pair run length matrix and the black-white-black combination run length matrix, are computed for each detected block. These matrices describe the occurrence of various black-white and black-white-black run lengths within blocks.

Three texture features, called short run emphasis, long run emphasis, and extra long run emphasis, are derived from these matrices and used in block classification based on linear discriminant functions.

PARAMETERS: More than 5 parameters have to be adjusted.

OUTPUT: Rectangular blocks classified as titles, paragraphs, line drawings, pictures.

PROCESSING TIME: It takes 2 (7.2) s for page segmentation and 0.6 (2.3) s for texture feature extraction and block classification when processing 100 (200) dpi images on a SUN 3/60.

ADVANTAGES: Quite fast on 100 dpi images, moderately fast on 200 dpi images.

DISADVANTAGES:
- Too many parameters to be tuned.
- Suitable only for rectangular layouts without skew.
- Greyscale images cannot be directly processed (prior binarisation is necessary).

2.2 Gabor filtering

To make the segmentation more robust to a document skew, a filter bank consisting of several orientation-selective 2-D Gabor filters is used to detect the texture features of text and non-text (background, pictures) components [6]. After that, these features are used for clustering the pixels into larger regions. This method is mainly designed to separate text and halftone pictures and it does not deal with binary line-drawings.

INPUT: Greyscale image of 75 dpi.
ALGORITHM:

Step 1. Apply the Gabor transform with different spatial frequencies and orientations.

Step 2. Compute the texture feature images.

Step 3. Cluster the feature vectors corresponding to each pixel.

Step 4 (Optional) Detect the connected components and find bounding boxes of the regions, if these regions are rectangles.

In step 1 the Gabor transform with m different spatial frequencies and p different orientations is applied to the original image by producing n=mp filtered images.

In the next step, each filtered image is first transformed with nonlinearity $(\tanh(\alpha t))$, and then a texture feature called the average absolute deviation is computed as the mean value in small overlapping windows centred at each pixel. The window size depends on the given spatial frequency. The values of each pixel in n feature images form an n-dimensional feature vector. These vectors are grouped into K clusters by using a squared-error clustering algorithm.

PARAMETERS: n (depends on application), $\alpha=0.25$, K (depends on application).

OUTPUT: Either bounding boxes around detected regions, if the document's layout consists of rectangular blocks, or a labelled bitmap where pixels belonging to the different classes have different labels.

PROCESSING TIME: It takes about 2 min to process a 512x512 image on a SUN SPARC 2.

ADVANTAGES: Skew-insensitive.

DISADVANTAGES: Too slow and very memory-consuming.

2.3 The texture co-occurrence spectrum technique

This technique [10] extracts information about the co-occurrence of pixel values within a window centred at each pixel.

INPUT: Binary or greyscale image.

ALGORITHM:

Step 1. Scan the image, pixel by pixel, and compute the feature vectors within a 5x5 window of each pixel.

Step 2. Extract the regions by applying the nearest neighbour classifier to the feature vectors.

The feature vector contains accumulated information extracted by four operators oriented at 0, 45, 90, and 135 degrees inside a 5x5 window. Each operator is applied to the four neighbours of the central pixel along a given direction.

PARAMETERS: None.

OUTPUT: Rectangular blocks.

PROCESSING TIME: Not reported.

ADVANTAGES:

- Can process both binary and greyscale images.
- No parameters to be set.

DISADVANTAGES: Designed to extract mainly rectangular blocks.

2.4 White tiles

This technique [2] segments and classifies an image based on white tiles or background spaces surrounding the document regions. This is in contrast to other approaches which rely on foreground information. White tiles provide a flexible data representation combining advantages of both rectangles (easy and fast access to pixels, simple description) and polygons (accurate representation of complex shaped and skewed regions), while avoiding their disadvantages (lack of efficiency in dealing with arbitrary layouts and page skew - for rectangles; difficult and time-consuming search for the data inside the regions - for polygons). Each tile represents the widest area of white space that can be represented by a rectangle.

INPUT: Binary image.

ALGORITHM:

Step 1. Segmentation using the white tiles.

Step 2. Classification based on texture features derived from white tiles.

The segmentation results in a net (array) of white tiles. Tracing through these tiles identifies the countour of each region and then textural features counting on the number, type (wide or narrow), and area of white tiles are employed for classification.

PARAMETERS: 4 thresholds should be predefined.

OUTPUT: Net (array) of white tiles together with classification labels for each region.

PROCESSING TIME: Not reported.

ADVANTAGES:

- Robust representation of complex shaped regions.
- Tolerant to significant skew.

DISADVANTAGES: Can only process binary images.

2.5 The neural network approach

A neural network approach to document classification is proposed in paper [7]. A two-layer neural network is trained with the backpropagation algorithm to obtain a moderate set of masks of MxM pixels which best discriminate between text, background, line-drawings and pictures, using sample data from these classes. Convolving these masks with the input image produces texture features used for classification of each image pixel by the neural network into one of three classes: text+line-drawings, halftone pictures, and background. The regions belonging to the first class are further binarised and a connected component analysis is applied for text/line-drawings separation. This method is robust to different languages, being able to discriminate text regions composed of such languages as English and Chinese, for example.

INPUT: Greyscale image of 100 dpi.

ALGORITHM:

Step 1. Learning the best discriminating masks.

Step 2. Convolving the input image with these masks.

Step 3. 3-class segmentation of the texture image.

Step 4. Postprocessing and separation of the text and line-drawing regions.

The purpose of step 1 is to select a moderate set of texture masks that minimises the classification error when discriminating halftones, background, and text+line-drawings in document images. The neural network used for learning these masks is a multilayer perceptron with 2 hidden layers. The backpropagation algorithm is employed to train the network with 1,000,000 randomly chosen samples of MxM pixels. Initially, the network topology is M^2x20x20x3. This means that the input layer contains M^2 nodes, two hidden layers consisting of 20 nodes each, and 3 nodes are in the output layer. A node saliency technique [8] prunes the number of nodes to 16 in the first hidden layer, which is equal to the number of the masks. The coefficients of the masks are weights of the connections between the nodes of the input and the first hidden layers.

The trained masks are convolved with the input image in order to obtain a texture image used in classification.

The classification into 3 classes is done on a 50 dpi subsampled image by applying the same network as used in the training, but now the network's topology is M^2x16x20x3. As a result, each pixel obtains a particular class label after this step.

A postprocessing step is necessary to remove small noisy elements and to merge the pixels into large regions. This operation is also done on a 50 dpi image. The image is first smoothed by analysing a 3x3 neighbourhood of each pixel and by assigning the central pixel's class label to the majority class of its neighbourhood. After that, the morphological operations are applied to merge together adjacent regions belonging to the same class. Finally, small components with an area of less than 10 pixels are assigned to the background. The regions of text+line-drawings are further binarised with a global threshold T_1 determined empirically and the connected component analysis is applied to separate text and line-drawings, where component size is used as criterion (if it exceeds a threshold T_2 on a 100 dpi image both in horizontal and vertical directions, then it is a line-drawing, otherwise text). Having obtained the large homogeneous regions and assuming that images consist of right rectangular blocks, bounding boxes are finally placed around each region.

PARAMETERS: M=7 pixels, T_1=150, T_2=46 pixels.

OUTPUT: Bounding boxes placed around detected regions.

PROCESSING TIME: It takes 35 s for classification using the neural network and 25-50 s for text/line drawings discrimination and postprocessing on a SUN SPARC 20 (original image sizes are 1080x780 pixels). This does not include the training time for the neural network which is not reported.

ADVANTAGES: Can discriminate text regions composed of different languages.

DISADVANTAGES: Quite slow and the size of the training set is enormous.

2.6 The multiscale technique with soft classification

In paper, [4] authors notice that document segmentation, if one considers it to be texture segmentation, becomes much more difficult than ordinary texture segmentation because of both large intra-class and inter-class variations in textural features. That is why they use multiscale analysis and extract features at different scales that are further classified with soft computing techniques. A priori knowledge about documents to be processed can be also incorporated into this method. The method is robust to unconstrained document layouts and page skew.

INPUT: Greyscale image of 200-300 dpi.
ALGORITHM:

Step 1. Neural network training with a conjugate gradient algorithm.

Step 2. Multiscale, wavelet packet analysis and texture feature extraction over small local windows.

Step 3. Classification of each window.

Step 4. Soft integration of local estimations.

Step 5. Contextual postprocessing.

The training set consists of 200 16x16 pixel samples from text, binary graphics, and halftone pictures. Examples of blocks containing the data of several classes are also included.

Wavelet packet analysis is chosen because of fast algorithms available for its computation, its flexibility to domain specific information, and perfect application to image compression. The low-order moments of wavelet packet components are used as texture features for classification of small local windows of MxM pixels.

Because the texture features computed over a region can contain information from more than one texture class, it is difficult to draw a sharp boundary between classes. A feed-forward multilayer neural network is used to classify the texture features computed over each local window. The topology of the network is 6x8x3 and the input nodes are linear, whereas the hidden and output nodes are sigmoid nonlinearities. The three outputs correspond to the votes associated with text, picture, and graphics classes and each output takes values in the range [0,1]. The 3-dimensional decision vector made up of these votes is a local classification for each window.

Decisions obtained over local windows are often uncertain and integration of several local decisions is therefore necessary, because several neighbouring windows tend to produce a more reliable result. The soft (fuzzy) decision vectors for each window are computed as a weighted sum of decision vectors obtained independently from neighbouring overlapping windows with a shift step of w pixels between the adjacent windows. Such computations involving several small windows are more accurate than those made over one larger window. The decision integration is done at several scales from low to high image resolution and within each scale as well. The final, still fuzzy decision about window class is based on the closeness of the top best class candidates.

The last step can facilitate further analysis, if a priori knowledge about the document and its structure is available. Examples of this knowledge are minimum/maximum font sizes, specific attributes on a page, such as page numbers, minimum distances between regions belonging to the different classes.

PARAMETERS: M=16, w=4.

OUTPUT: Labelled set of windows.

PROCESSING TIME: It takes 18 s for feature extraction and 4 s for their classification on a SUN SPARC 20 with the parameters M and w given above and the image resolution of 300 dpi.

ADVANTAGES:
- Robust to skew and different document layouts.
- Moderately fast.

DISADVANTAGES: Extra processing is necessary to combine the classified windows into larger regions.

2.7 The Hidden Markov Model (HMM) approach

Text detection on a textured background is an issue of paper [3]. The method consists of three steps: texture feature extraction by using Laws' masks, coarse segmentation to detect the candidates for text regions, and fine segmentation within these candidate regions to separate text from textured background.

INPUT: Greyscale image.

ALGORITHM:

Step 1. Training HMMs with the number of states N.

Step 2. Texture feature extraction.

Step 3. Block-based coarse segmentation.

Step 4. Pixel-based fine segmentation.

Stationary HMMs (their number is equal to L and it depends on the number of texture classes) are used; one model for each texture type and each model is trained independently of the others with the Baum-Welch algorithm. That is, if a new texture class is added, a new model is created and trained individually only on samples of this class in contrast to many neural networks, where a complete network's retraining is necessary for samples of all classes in this case.

To compute the texture features, 4 5x5 pixel Laws' masks are applied one by one to the image and each pixel is represented by a sequence of length 8 (due to 8 rotations of each mask in 45 degrees) with each element of the sequence being a vector of 4x1 (due to 4 masks).

The purpose of the coarse segmentation is to quickly locate the candidate regions for text. The image is first divided into 8x8 non-overlapping blocks, then a 3x3 neighbourhood (which includes 8 blocks) of each block is analysed. Each of the eight neighbours of the block in question is labelled by employing the pretrained N-state HMMs. The central block belongs to a particular class, if all its 8 neighbours belong to the same class, otherwise it is assigned to fuzzy (boundary between text and background) blocks. The candidates for text are pure text blocks and fuzzy blocks which are further processed in the next step.

The fine segmentation aims at more accurate segmentation and extraction of the text data and it involves computations at pixel level. A square window centred at a given pixel is split into 4 3x3 subwindows and a concept of the maximum likelihood probability is used for each subwindow in order to label the central pixel.

PARAMETERS: L (depends on the number of texture classes), $N \in \{4,6,8\}$.

OUTPUT: Labelled bitmap.

PROCESSING TIME: Not reported.

ADVANTAGES:
- Text extraction on a complex textured background.
- Easy adaptation to new texture classes.

DISADVANTAGES: Seems to be time and memory consuming.

3 Discussion

We shall now briefly consider some important features of the aforementioned methods. The documents processed are magazines and newspapers. Almost all methods assume that the image background is white except for Chen's paper [3] where it is textured. Most of the methods are designed to process either greyscale or binary images. We did not find any references to colour images.

The texture-based layout analysis methods can be divided into two groups. The methods of the first group (Group 1) compute textural features over a given window whose sizes are MxM pixels, where M is much less than the image size [3,4,7,10]. This can be done in two ways. With the first way, the image is scanned pixel by pixel such that the neighbouring windows are overlapped and each pixel obtains its class label. According to the second way, the image is divided into a number of small usually non-overlapping windows and the label is assigned to each window. This means that the document regions are extracted after window/pixel classification. The methods of the second group (Group 2), on the other hand, first extract the regions and then each region is classified by using a number of texture features [2,12].

Postprocessing is often necessary for methods of Group 1 in order to merge the pixels or windows into larger regions. The methods of Group 1 are more robust (due to local processing) to different layouts and/or document skew than the methods of Group 2, where region extraction procedures result in more or less strict restictions on the document skew and layout.

Problems that are not often considered by the methods of either group are big character detection and extraction of small text components inside graphics. Big characters can appear in document titles and headings or as drop caps (the first letters at the beginning of the first paragraph). Text embedded in graphics can be found, for example, in flow charts or plots. The first problem seems to be difficult for both groups because of misclassification (either the whole drop cap or some of its parts can be easily classified as picture or graphics). The second problem is somehow easier for methods belonging to Group 1 because they will not merge text and surrounding graphics as will probably happen by applying methods from Group 2, where image "smearing" is often used to obtain the regions.

The computational complexity of all methods is quite high (processing time depends on image sizes and resolution). This is because of pixel-based computations, large image sizes, and the high complexity of the texture analysis methods normally used. Image sizes of 2,500x3,300 pixels are typical in document processing. Therefore, such techniques as Gabor filters used in ordinary texture analysis, are computationally very expensive. The computational complexity also depends on whether adjacent windows are overlapped or not when a method of this type is applied. The overlapped windows usually lead to more accurate localisation of block boundaries at the cost of the processing time.

A supervised learning of texture classes cannot embrace all real cases because of a large variety of different textures that document images usually have. This is the main distinction from ordinary texture segmentation and classification, where the number of classes is often known or small.

In principle, the document layout analysis methods classified as non-texture-based are capable of doing the same and have similar features (see, for example, papers [1,5,9,11]) as the texture-based techniques. Texture-based methods seem to be better in certain cases. Examples of applications where the non-texture-based methods tend to fail are text extraction on a complex textured background [3] and separation of regions containing a text of different languages [7]. The latter case is very important because it facilitates text segmentation and OCR. As indicated in paper [3], the texture-based methods are less limited to a specific document layout and page skew because in this case the segmentation only relies on analysis of a local neighbourhood of a pixel.

Finally, we consider situations where texture-based methods may not be useful. It seems that colour document image processing (WWW pages, CD and book covers, and video) is one area because of the very complex nature of colour images in combination with noise and special design effects. The texture-based methods will also be hardly advantageous over their non-texture counterparts for upright document images with a zero skew and/or with a simple layout because in this case they often need extra processing to obtain the large regions, which implies extra processing time.

4 Conclusion

This paper contains a brief overview of document layout analysis methods where the problem is considered as texture segmentation and classification. These methods can be classified into two groups (Group 1 and Group 2). The methods of Group 1 are more robust to different layouts and document skew than the methods of Group 2. Moreover, some of the methods in Group 1 can be used for text extraction on a complex textured background and for language separation. These are tasks that are very difficult for methods of Group 2 and for non-texture-based methods as well. Problems that ought to be solved are the high computational complexity of layout analysis methods and proper detection of drop caps and text embedded in graphics.

Acknowledgements

The financial support provided by the Technology Development Center of Finland is gratefully acknowledged.

References

1. T. Akiyama and N. Hagita, Automated entry system for printed documents, *Patt. Rec.* **23**, 1141–1154 (1990).
2. A. Antonacopoulos and R.T. Ritchings, Representation and classification of complex-shaped printed regions using white tiles, *Proc. of 3rd ICDAR*, 1132–1135 (1995).
3. J.-L. Chen, A simplified approach to the HMM based texture analysis and its application to document segmentation, *Patt. Rec. Lett.* **18**, 993–1007 (1997).
4. K. Etemad *et al*, Multiscale segmentation of unstructured document pages using soft decision integration, *IEEE Trans. on PAMI* **19**, 92–96 (1997).
5. F. Hönes and J. Lichter, Layout extraction of mixed mode documents, *Machine Vision and Applications* **7**, 237–246 (1994).
6. A.K. Jain and S. Bhattacharjee, Text segmentation using Gabor filters for automatic document processing, *Machine Vision and Applications* **5**, 169–184 (1992).
7. A.K. Jain and Y. Zhong, Page segmentation using texture analysis, *Patt. Rec.* **29**, 743–770 (1996).
8. J. Mao and A.K. Jain. Texture classification and segmentation using multiresolution simultaneous autoregressive models, *Patt. Rec.* **25**, 173–188 (1992).
9. T. Pavlidis and H. Zhou, Page segmentation and classification, *Comp. Vision, Graph., and Image Proc.* **54**, 484–496 (1992).
10. J.S. Payne *et al*, Document segmentation using texture analysis, *Proc. of 12th ICPR*, 380–382 (1994).
11. J. Sauvola and M. Pietikäinen, Page segmentation and classification using fast feature extraction and connectivity analysis, *Proc. of 3rd ICDAR*, 1127–1131 (1995).
12. D. Wang and S.N. Srihari, Classification of newspaper image blocks using texture analysis, *Comp. Vision, Graph., and Image Proc.* **47**, 327–352 (1989).

TONGUE TEXTURE ANALYSIS USING GABOR WAVELET OPPONENT COLOUR FEATURES FOR TONGUE DIAGNOSIS IN TRADITIONAL CHINESE MEDICINE

PONG C YUEN, *Z Y KUANG, *W WU and Y T WU

Department of Computer Science
Hong Kong Baptist University, Hong Kong

*Guangzhou University of Traditional Chinese Medicine
Guangzhou, China

Email: pcyuen@comp.hkbu.edu.hk

Abstract

This article reports an application of using Gabor Wavelet Opponent Colour Features (GWOCF) for tongue diagnosis in Traditional Chinese Medicine (TCM). This project focuses on the standardization of the tongue diagnosis in TCM. The objective is to develop a set of quantitative measurement for tongue diagnosis using computer vision techniques. To achieve this goal, we propose to use GWOCF for determining different types of tongue proper and tongue coating textures from a tongue image. Two experiments are presented. In the first experiment, GWOCF is directly extracted from tongue image for recognition. In the second experiment, we employ colour information to pre-classify the known texture image before extracting GWOCF. 63 tongue images captured from 63 patients in Guangzhou University of Traditional Chinese Medicine's hospital are used for testing. It is found that with colour pre-classification process, 89% of recognition accuracy can be achieved. This is a revised version of our conference paper in [12].

Keywords: Tongue diagnosis, Traditional Chinese Medicine, Texture Analysis, Gabor Wavelet opponent colour features

1. Introduction

Traditional Chinese Medicine (TCM) has been developed for over thousands of years and is an important component of Chinese culture. The basic principles of TCM are based on the four techniques of diagnosis [1], namely inspection, auscultation-olfaction, inquiry and palpation. The inspection process includes the inspection of body, tongue, excreta. Auscultation-olfaction process is to collect the information from speech, respiration, cough, hiccup and eructation. Inquiry process

179

is to obtain patient's general information through questioning. The palpation process is to check the patient's pulse. Most of the TCM theories are qualitative and there is not sufficient quantitative measurement. In turn, the quality of the TCM practitioners highly depend on their personal experience. To set up a scientific and systematic TCM system, we have to develop a set of quantitative measurement from the traditional theories.

Tongue diagnosis is an important part among the four techniques of diagnosis, which have been reported in many Chinese medicine literatures [1]. Tongue diagnosis focuses on the tongue proper and its coating. The tongue proper is composed of muscles, vessels and tissue, while its coating is a layer of mossy substance on its surface produced by stomach. A brief description on the tongue diagnosis in TCM is given in Section 2. In short, the objective of this project is to,

➢   define a set of standard and objective measurement for tongue diagnosis; and accordingly,
➢   translate existing qualitative measurement into quantitative measurement.

The use of image processing approach for tongue diagnosis for Traditional Chinese Medicine (TCM) has been started in mid 80s. Researches in this area are mainly done in China and Taiwan. There are a lot of research articles on tongue diagnosis for TCM, mostly from medical point of view. However, only five articles for tongue diagnosis using image processing approach have been published. Also, no tongue diagnosis research article can be found outside China. Coincidentally, the main objective of these three articles is to standardize the tongue diagnosis for TCM. Below is a brief review on the five articles.

Suen et al. [7] first reported a study on tongue analysis using image processing and pattern recognition technique by computer. This article suggested using colour information to distinguish different types of tongue proper and tongue coating colour. Although the results of this paper are quite primitive, it provides a good direction for this research area. Along Suen et al.'s direction, Zhao et al. [8] developed an algorithm, which is able to recognize three types of tongue proper colour and five types of tongue coating colour. They employed the RGB colour space for the analysis. In 1994, Yu et al. [9] developed a computer vision system for tongue diagnosis. The system includes a hardware platform with an Intel 80286 microprocessor and an image capturing system. The recognition rate is 86.34% in classifying four types of tongues, namely, light read tongue, dark red tongue, purplish red tongue and dark purple tongue. A clustering technique on the colour component of the RGB space is used. Chiu et al. [5] proposed a structural recognition approach for tongue diagnosis. This method adopted the RGB model for mapping the tongue colours to some known categories and then employed traditional texture algorithms, such as spatial gray dependency matrices [10] and Fourier power spectrum [11] for texture analysis. The improvement of this system was reported in [6] by quantizing the chromatic and textural properties of tongue. Chiu proposed a good direction by applying texture algorithm to analyse tongue texture. However, when analyzing the texture, the colour information is not considered.

This article proposes to apply the Gabor Wavelet opponents colour features [2] (GWOCF) for tongue texture analysis. GWOCF contains both the multi-channel frequency properties and colour features, in which the accuracy in extracting tongue features is increased.

2. Background of Tongue diagnosis in TCM

Tongue diagnosis is the mandatory and important step in the traditional Chinese Medicine (TCM). In TCM theory [1], tongue is the window of heart. The spleen reflects itself on the tongue. As the tongue is connected with a number of viscera via the meridians, the essential of the viscera can ascend to nourish the tongue and pathological processes are also reflected on it. Therefore observing the tongue can help diagnosis pathological changes of the viscera. Tongue diagnosis has a very long history and has been established as a systematic TCM theory.

Tongue diagnosis focuses on the tongue proper and its coating. The tongue proper is composed of muscles, vessels and tissue, while its coating is a layer of mossy substance on its surface produced by stomach. In TCM theory, they examine the colour and texture of both tongue proper and tongue coating. Based on these tongue features, a preliminary conclusion can be made. For example, a yellowish coating and a red dry tongue are often seen in endogenous pathogenic heat due to excess, while a white coating and a light-coloured and moist tongue are often seen in endogenous pathogenic cold due to deficiency [1]. According to the TCM literature [1] [5] (most of them are in Chinese), the description on tongue diagnosis is shown in Figure 1. As shown in Figure 1, we need to extract texture and colour features for both tongue proper and tongue coating. The analysis of the tongue's movement is beyond the scope of this project.

3. Gabor Wavelet Opponent Colour Features

Many texture analysis techniques have been developed in the last twenty years. Multi-channel filtering is one of the promising approaches and Gabor Wavelet [3] provides very good results on multi-channel filtering in Fourier domain. Most of the existing texture analysis techniques focused on the gray level images. However, the tongue texture to be analyzed contains colour information. One way is to discard the colour information and transform the colour image into gray intensity. This is not a good approach as the colour information is lost and the tongue textures are quite similar. Therefore, we adopt the colour opponent features [4]. By combining the Gabor Wavelet and colour opponent features, Gabor Wavelet colour opponent features can be constructed.

In this paper, a bank of real circularly symmetric Gabor filters [3] is employed and defined as follows.

where m is the index for the scale and n is the index for the orientation.

$$f_{mn}(x,y) = \frac{1}{2\pi\sigma_m^2}\exp\left\{-\frac{x^2+y^2}{2\sigma_m^2}\right\} \times \cos(2\pi(u_m x\cos\theta_n + u_n y\sin\theta_n)) \qquad (1)$$

The opponent feature [2] is defined as

$$\Psi_{ijmm'n} = \sqrt{\left(\sum d_{ijmm'n}^2(x,y)\right)} \qquad (2)$$

where $d_{ijmm'n}$ is the difference of the normalized filter images of different Gabor wavelet spectral band i and j.

4. Experimental Results

The image acquisition setup in the hospital is shown in Figure 2. A 3-CCD digital camera is used to capture the tongue image in order to minimize the colour distortion. A sample tongue image is shown in Figure 3 (colour image). The reference textures (colour) are shown in Figure 4 and the size of each reference texture is 36x36.

For a tongue image to be analyzed, the image is divided into a number of blocks, each block of the size 36x36 as shown in Figure 5. The tongue region is manually selected while the non-tongue blocks are removed. All the non-tongue blocks in Figure 3 are removed and the tongue region is zoomed in as shown in Figure 5. Each block in tongue region is called as *tongue texture block* (TTB). For each TTB, the following distance measurement [2] is performed.

$$d_{ij} = \sum_{k=1}^{q}\left(\frac{f_k^i - f_k^j}{\sigma(f_i)}\right)^2 \qquad (3)$$

where $\sigma(f_i)$ is the standard deviation of f_i over all the reference textures.

In both experiments, a three scale and four orientation filter bank is defined and a total of 36 unichrome features are computed for three spectral bands [2]. Also 84 opponent features are computed. Therefore, a total of 120 features are used for classification.

Figure 1 shows that the tongue proper texture includes thorny, cracked and indented while enlarged and thin are used to describe the shape of tongue. The tongue coating textures include thickness, moisture, viscosity and peeling. This paper concentrates on detecting five types of textures, namely, thorny, cracked, thin coating, thick coating and no coating. Although we are going to detect only five types of textures, all these five types of textures may have different colour such as white, yellow, pale yellow, dark, red, pale red etc, as shown in Figure 1. Therefore, there are 96 types of texture as shown in Figure 4 when colour information is considered.

63 tongue images from 63 patients are used for evaluating the capability of the proposed method. The images are captured with two different camera settings at different time. 32 images are captured in an automatic mode of the CCD camera. Another 31 images are captured with longer exposure time so that the average gray level intensity of the second batch of images is higher than that in the first batch. Although each tongue image is captured in fixed distance, the size of the tongue may have much variation because of the physical tongue size are actually different for each patient. So the number of blocks in each tongue image varies from 50 TTBs to 180 TTBs. Therefore, more than 7,000 testing TTBs are used for evaluation. The accuracy is measured by the following formula [6].

$$Accuracy = \frac{Number\ of\ correct\ classified\ TTBs}{Total\ number\ of\ TTBs} x100\% \qquad (4)$$

Two experiments are reported in this section. In the first experiment, all the reference textures are used for determining the characteristic of each 36x36 TTB in tongue image. The recognition accuracy for experiment 1 is 72%. In the second experiment, the reference textures are pre-classified into three subsets based on the normalized RGB colour. In determining the texture in each TTB, the TTB is pre-classified based on its normalized RGB values. The accuracy is increased to 89% (in both experiments, the correct match of TTB is based on human judgement).

We have also developed an interactive software application in Windows 95 platform. User can select a 36x36 block from a tongue image. The colour and the tongue texture characteristics will be determined automatically. The user interface is shown in Figure 6.

5. Conclusions

We have successfully applied Gabor Wavelet opponent colour features in the tongue diagnosis for traditional Chinese medicine. It is also found that if the unknown tongue texture block (TTB) is pre-classified based on its colour information, the recognition accuracy is increased dramatically. Comparing with the existing work on tongue diagnosis, the proposed method provides better performance because colour information is considered. It is also shown the accuracy is increased.

As the final goal of this project is to develop a set of standard and objective measurement for tongue diagnosis, the accuracy results are not sufficient. The further development of this project will be concentrated on the following issues.

- Colour pre-classification;
- Other texture analysis algorithms for representing tongue textures
- Reduce the computational load and improve the accuracy

Moreover, most of the tongue features are overlapped on the feature space. It is not a good method to select only a few representatives from the tongue images for representing that kind of feature. In addition, traditional clustering algorithm may not work in this application. In turn, we will also concentrate on the development of a new clustering method. Finally, a tongue image may contain more than one unique tongue proper and coating features. Therefore, in evaluating the correctness of the matching, it is also a hard thing to do. The main problem is that we do not have a ground true to evaluate the features of TTB.

Conclusively speaking, the results of this approach are encouraging. Towards this direction, the standardization of tongue diagnosis can be achieved in coming years.

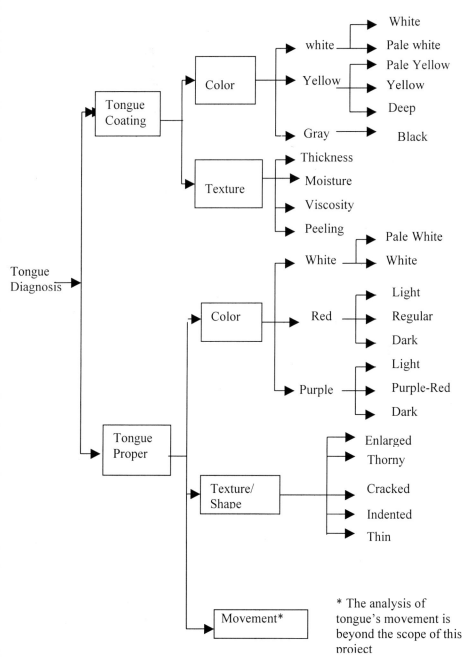

Figure 1: Characteristics of tongue for tongue diagnosis in TCM

Acknowledgment

This project was supported by the Faculty Research Grant, Hong Kong Baptist University. The authors would like to thanks Dr. C H Li for useful discussions, Mr. K C Woo for implementing and testing of algorithms, and Mr. James Yuen for developing the software package in Windows 95 platform. Finally, the authors would also thank Ms. Joan Yuen for proofreading this manuscript.

References

1. H Yiu, *Fundamental of Traditional Chinese Medicine*, Foreign Language Press, Beijing, 1992.
2. A Jain and G Healey, "A multiscale representation including opponent colour features for texture recognition", *IEEE Trans. On Image Processing*, Vol. 7, No. 1, pp. 124 – 128, 1998.
3. A K Jain and F Farrokhnia, "Unsupervised texture segmentation using Gabor filters", *Pattern Recognition*, Vol. 24, pp. 1167-1186, 1991.
4. L M Hurvich and D Jameson, "An opponent-process theory of colour vision", *Physiol Rev.* Vol. 64, pp. 384-404, 1957.
5. C C Chiu, H S Lin and S L Lin, "A structural texture recognition approach for medical diagnosis through tongue", *Biomedical Engineering – Application, Basis and Communications,* Vol. 7, No. 2, pp. 11-16, 1995.
6. C C Chiu, "The development of a computerized tongue diagnosis system*", Biomedical Engineering – Application, Basis and Communications*, Vol. 8, No. 4, pp. 342-349, 1996.
7. L Sun, Z Cheng, F Gao, H Xie and W Xia, "Research on standardization of tongue diagnosis using image processing", *Chinese Medicine letters*, Vo. 5, No.4, pp. 5-7, 1986. (in Chinese).
8. R Zhao, B Wei, R Ding, P Guo, X Zhen, S Xu, Z Huang and H Gao, "Description and classification of tongue texture and coating*", Chinese Medicine Magazine*, No.2, pp. 47-48, 1989 (in Chinese).
9. X Yu, Y Tan, Z Zhu, Z Suo, G Jin, W Weng, X Xu and W Ge, "Research on automatic tongue diagnosis", *Biomedical Engineering letters*, Vol. 13, No, 4, pp. 336-343, 1994 (in Chinese).
10. R M Haralick, K Shanmugan and I Dinstien, "Texture features for image classification", *IEEE Trans. On System, Man and Cybernetics*, Vol.3, No. 6, 1973.
11. R C Gonzalez and R E Woods, *Digital image processing*, Addison Wesley, 1992.

12. P C Yuen, Z Y Kuang, W Wu and Y T Wu, "Tongue texture analysis using opponent colour features for tongue diagnosis in traditional Chinese medicine", Proceeding of *International Workshop on Texture Analysis in Machine Vision*, pp. 21 - 27, 1999

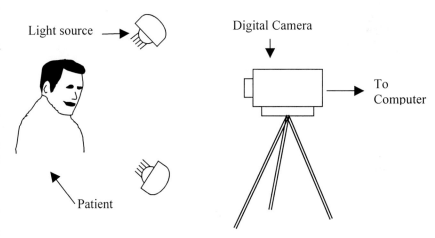

Figure 2: Image acquisition Setup

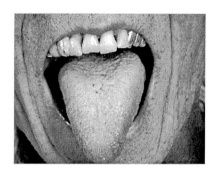

Figure 3: Tongue Image (colour)

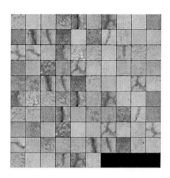

Figure 4: Reference Textures

TTB

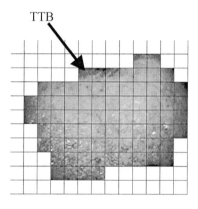

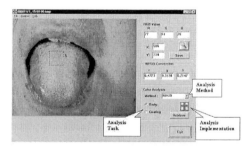

Figure 5: Selected TTBs to be analyzed   Figure 6: A tongue diagnosis interface

TEXTURE ANALYSIS OF X-RAY IMAGES FOR DETECTION OF CHANGES IN BONE MASS AND STRUCTURE

A. MATERKA AND P. CICHY

Institute of Electronics, Technical University of Łódź, Stefanowskiego 18, 90-924 Łódź, Poland, E-mail: materka@ck-sg.p.lodz.pl

J. TULISZKIEWICZ

Polish Mother Memorial Hospital Institute, Rzgowska 281, 93-338 Łódź, Poland

An attempt is made to apply digital image analysis techniques to the evaluation of bone mass and internal structure, based on X-ray images. Images of distal forearm bone are investigated. A calibration phantom is included in the image to equalize the image intensity. Both raw and equalized images are analyzed and results are compared. A number of first-order texture parameters and fractal dimensions are evaluated. These texture-derived image features are correlated with the bone mineral density estimated by means of dual-photonabsorptiometry (DXA), a standard diagnostic technique. The effect of image blur and noise on texture parameters is investigated as well, showing significant influence of image distortion on fractal features, and thus indicating the need for image preprocessing before texture analysis.

1. Introduction

There is a growing interest during the last decades in finding effective diagnostic methods for skeletal system diseases. Among these diseases, the osteoporosis is characterized by changes in bone mass density and structure that make the bone susceptible to fracture. Finding efficient means of preventing this disease, which affects primarily middle-aged and elderly people, is of growing importance to modern society whose average population age increases constantly. One of the techniques used for skeletal system diagnosis is standard X-ray examination [3] that allows detection of changes not only in the outer – compact part of the bone, but also changes in the inner – spongy bone microarchitecture.

The advantages of the X-ray technique are common availability and low cost; however, interpretation of radiograms is not an easy task. It is estimated that by means of traditional X-ray analysis, changes related to calcium decrease can be noticed at 30-60% loss of the bone mass, which corresponds to an already advanced phase of the disease [3,11]. Other examination techniques, such as densitometry, CT tomography and magnetic resonance imaging require expensive equipment. They are then of limited availability to a gross population of patients. There is a need for an inexpensive and simple diagnostic technique that would allow detection of early changes in the structure and mass density of the bone. Such a method would be very useful for prevention of the skeletal system diseases as well as for their treatment in a non-developed phase. It is postulated in this paper that texture analysis of digitized X-ray images can be considered as an alternative to standard techniques of skeletal system diagnosis.

At present, the only method widely accepted by physicians, that is able to detect a decreased mass of the bone (which is the most important risk factor for osteoporosis) is densitometry [9,1]. The most popular densitometric technique, of high accuracy and sensitivity, is dual-energy X-ray absorpiometry DXA [12]. This technique has been utilized in this paper as a reference method.

2. Materials

X-ray images of forearm distal bone were taken for a group of 50 subjects of different age. The same persons were measured the forearm bone mineral density using DXA. The X-ray images were all taken at 53 kV and 4 mAs, and films were developed using the same chemical process. A calibration phantom Agfa Mamoray of specified absorption of X-ray radiation was placed in each image. The images were digitized at 7 bits/pixel using a CCD camera. The digital images were brightness-standardized by making the phantom average brightness the same in all images. A 256×256-pixel region of interest (ROI) was defined in the field of every image (Fig. 1). The image texture within the ROI was characterized by means of texture statistical parameters and image surface fractal dimensions, as described in the next section.

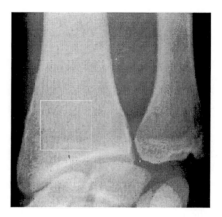

Figure 1. Example of an X-ray image of distal forearm bone with a square ROI.

Figure 2 shows examples of ROI images that correspond to bones of different values of bone mineral density (BMD). One can notice the gradual brightness decrease and bone microarchitecture degradation with the reduced contents of calcium.

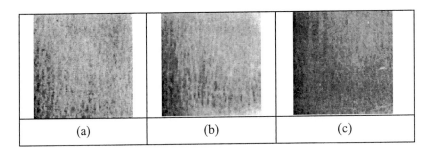

Figure 2. Sample X-ray images of bone tissue for different BMD coefficients
(a) BMD = 0.56 g/cm², (b) BMD = 0.31 g/cm², (c) BMD = 0.14 g/cm².

3. Methods

The reference method in our study is DXA densitometry, implemented using a Lunar DPX instrument at Polish Mother Memorial Hospital Institute, Lodz, Poland. To reduce the influence of the soft tissue on the analysis results, dual energy radiation was used, of respectively 38 keV and 70 keV. The Lunar DPX instrument allows measuring the distal forearm bone in a region 140×126 mm, using 117 scanning lines, each of 210 points. It is then a low-resolution examination. It lasts typically 5 min and the dose absorbed is less that 0.3 mrem. The *in vivo* accuracy is better that 1.5 %, with repeatability of 1 % [12].

First- and higher-order statistical parameters are often used to characterize image texture [6,11]. In this study, a number of image histogram-derived ROI parameters were investigated, including sample mean, standard deviation, skewness, kurtosis, energy and entropy. The complexity and self-similarity of texture at different scales are described by fractal dimension [8,5,7,10,4,2] which was also computed in the present work. From the variety of different methods of computing the fractal dimension, two techniques based respectively on Fourier transform and local image variance were employed that were simple to implement numerically. The FFT-derived fractal dimension was computed separately for vertical and horizontal direction. The image texture features were calculated using dedicated subroutines written in Matlab 5.2 language for a Pentium 120 MHz PC computer.

4. Results

Altogether, 50 X-ray bone images were digitally recorded. The images represented forearm bones of different BMD level that was independently measured for each subject by means of the DXA technique. Based on the densitometry results, the whole group of subjects was divided into 3 categories: normal – 19 subjects, of physiological loss of calcium (osteopenia) – 21 subjects, and of abnormal loss of calcium (osteoporosis) – 10 subjects. For every texture parameter, its mean and standard deviation were computed within each of the three groups of patients. Linear correlation coefficient with the bone mineral density was computed for every parameter and for all subjects. The statistical significance of the correlation was also evaluated. Table 1 shows results obtained for brightness-corrected images.

Table 1. Texture parameter statistics
T-score – result of DXA examination (difference to population BMD mean of young people, normalized to standard deviation), μ(σ) - mean value (standard deviation) of a given parameter, BMD – bone mineral density, μI – image mean, SDI – image standard deviation, sk – skewness, k - kurtosis, E - energy, Ent - entropy, FDv (FDh) – fractal dimension in vertical (horizontal) direction, FDvar- fractal dimension computed using variance method, *) p<0.005.

# sub-jects	T- score		BMD g/cm²	μI	SDI	sk	k	E	Ent	FDv	FDh	FDvar
19	sd> -1	μ	0.39	62.28	5.67	-0.32	-0.35	0.05	4.46	2.51	2.39	2.17
		σ	0.10	14.94	1.63	0.31	0.15	0.01	0.41	0.05	0.01	0.16
21	-1≥sd >-2.5	μ	0.32	50.24	4.13	-0.19	-0.33	0.08	3.98	2.56	2.41	2.32
		σ	0.06	9.29	0.15	0.33	0.42	0.00	0.03	0.04	0.02	0.22
10	sd≤ -2.5	μ	0.25	46.31	3.72	0.17	1.23	0.09	3.83	2.59	2.43	2.34
		σ	0.11	10.21	2.34	0.40	0.41	0.04	0.76	0.25	0.14	0.24
50	total	μ	0.33	54.05	4.63	-0.17	-0.03	0.07	4.13	2.55	2.40	2.27
		σ	0.06	8.89	1.46	0.33	2.2	0.03	0.49	0.08	0.06	0.19
		R		0.79	0.55	-0.57	-0.25	-0.51	0.54	-0.49	-0.36	-0.43
		p-value		1e-11 *	4e-5 *	3e-6 *	0.08	1e-4 *	5e-5 *	3e-4 *	0.01	1e-3 *

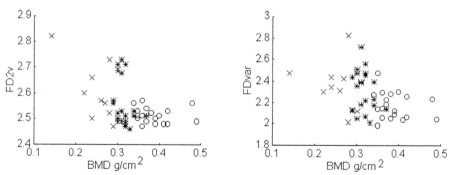

Figure 3. Image mean and standard deviation relationship to bone mineral density.

Figure 3 demonstrates the relationship between the bone mineral density and selected texture parameters of X-ray images, whereas Fig. 4 shows correlation between BMD and fractal dimension. The data obtained for different groups of subjects are distinguished graphically using 'o' for normal subjects (sd > -1), '*' for physiological loss of calcium (-1 ≥ sd ≥ -2.5), and 'x' for lowest-density bones (sd <

-2.5), where sd is the T-score (Lunar 1993). Table 2 shows the differences in the results of statistical texture analysis obtained for raw images and phantom-brightness-corrected images. The table contains also the values of linear correlation coefficient between the BMD and raw-image texture parameters and the results of t-test for correlation coefficients.

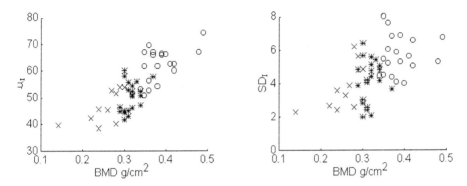

Figure 4. Fractal dimensions as functions of bone mineral density.

Table 2. Comparison of raw and brightness-corrected images
(*Δ denotes differences between feature values obtained for standardized and non-standardized images, R0 – correlation with BMD for raw images*)

# sub-jects	T-score		BMD g/cm²	ΔμI	ΔSDI	Δsk	Δk	ΔE	ΔEnt	ΔFDv	ΔFDh	ΔFD var
19	sd>-1	μ	0.39	11.07	-0.03	-0.02	-0.01	0.00	0.00	-0.01	-0.01	0.00
21	-1≥sd >-2.5	μ	0.32	11.75	0.10	0.01	-0.01	0.00	0.05	-0.03	-0.02	0.00
10	sd≤ -2.5	μ	0.25	15.06	-0.04	-0.03	-0.12	0.00	0.00	-0.01	-0.01	0.00
50		μ	0.33	12.63	-0.01	0.01	-0.05	0.00	-0.02	-0.02	-0.01	0.00
		R0	0.61	0.53	-0.47	-0.24	-0.50	0.53	-0.46	-0.38	-0.43	
		|R-R0|	0.18	0.02	0.10	0.01	0.02	0.01	0.03	0.01	0.00	
		p	2e-6 *	5e-5 *	4e-3 *	0.08	2e-4 *	6e-5 *	9e-4 *	6e-3 *	1e-3 *	

5. Discussion

Based on analysis of the linear correlation coefficient, one can state that there is a significant correlation between the bone mineral density measured by the standard DXA technique and the image mean, standard deviation, skewness, kurtosis, energy, entropy, fractal dimension in vertical dimension, and variance-based fractal dimension.

The fractal dimension reflects roughness of the bone image texture that is related to the bone microarchitecture (Fig. 2). It is of high importance, because mechanical endurance of the bone tissue depends largely on the state of the bone internal structure. For a subject suffering from osteoporosis (BMD = 0.14 g/cm^2, T-score = -6.63), high values of fractal dimension in the vertical direction (FDv = 2.82) and in the horizontal direction (FDh = 2.55) were obtained. The values of fractal dimension are lower for healthy subjects in this study (Table 1). Differences between the fractal dimensions in horizontal and vertical directions reflect the anisotropy of the image texture (Fig. 2).

Image brightness shows the highest correlation to BMD ($r = 0.79$, $p < 0.005$). This can be explained by the fact that lower calcium contents results in lower attenuation of X-rays in the bone, so the photographic film becomes darker and digital image brightness is reduced. This applies to brightness-equalized images. It is evident that image brightness standardization is a necessary preprocessing step for reliable analysis of image texture. The significance of this step is illustrated in Table 2. Correlation of image mean and skewness are significantly affected by a lack of brightness standardization. The other statistical parameters do not show much dependence on standardization, and the FDvar fractal dimension shows complete invariance to it.

One can conclude that by measuring changes in statistical texture parameters and fractal dimensions of X-ray images it is possible to monitor changes in calcium contents and internal structure of the bone. Texture analysis shows potential usefulness as an aid to the diagnosis of skeletal diseases. This initial research was carried out using first-order texture features only. Further work is needed to select optimum texture parameters from a variety of known approaches, including wavelet analysis and mathematical morphology derived features. It has been demonstrated also that there exist a degrading effect of image blur and noise, typical to X-ray images, on texture parameters. There is a need to elaborate techniques to reduce these effects, which is the subject of the current study. Also, high-resolution flat bed transparency scanner is being used at present for image digitization with an increased accuracy compared to the CCD camera. First experiments show that fractal dimensions computed for scanned radiographic films demonstrate significantly higher correlation to BMD compared with CCD-recorded images.

6 Acknowledgements

This work was performed within the framework of COST B11 European project. The authors appreciate the help of the staff of Department of Radiology A, Polish Mother Memorial Hospital Institute, Łódź, Poland, in collecting X-ray images and making DXA measurements.

References

1. Badurski J., Sawicki A. and Boczoń S., *Osteoporosis* (Osteoprint, Bialystok, 1994, in Polish).
2. Chan K., Quantitative characterization of electron micrograph image using fractal features, *IEEE Transactions on Biomedical Engineering* **42**, 10 (1995) pp. 1033-1037.
3. Czekalski S., Hoszowski K., Lorenc R., Walecki J., Miazgowski T., and Morawska J., Detection of osteoporosis, *Polski Tygodnik Lekarski* **XLVIII**, 3, XI (1993) pp. 46-49.
4. Dubuisson M., Dubes R., Efficacy of fractal features in segmentation images of natural textures, *Pattern Recognition Letters* **15** (1994) pp. 419-431.
5. Fortin C., Kumaresan K., Ohley W. and Hoefer R., Fractal dimension in the analysis of medical images, *IEEE Engineering in Medicine and Biology* (June 1992) pp. 65-71.
6. Haralick R., Statistical and structural approaches to texture, *Proceedings IEEE* **67**, 5 (1979) pp. 786-804.
7. Peitgen H., Jurgens H. and Saupe D., *Fractals for the Classroom* (Springer Verlag, New York, 1992).
8. Pentland A., Fractal-based description of natural scenes, *IEEE Transactions on Pattern Analysis and Machine Intelligence* **6**, 6 (1984) pp. 661-674.
9. Pluskiewicz W. and Rogala E., *Osteoporoza* (Śląska Akademia Medyczna, Katowice, 1996, in Polish).
10. Ruttiman U., Webber R. and Hazeirig J., Fractal dimension from radiographs of peridental alveolar bone. A possible diagnostic indicator of osteoporosis, *Oral Surg Oral Med Oral Pathol* **74**, 1 (1992) pp. 98-110.
11. Southard T. and Southard K., Detection of simulated osteoporosis in maxillae using radiographic texture analysis, *IEEE Transactions on Biomedical Engineering* **43**, 2 (1996) pp. 123-132.
12. Technical Manual, Lunar DPX, Documentation 8/93.

FEATURE EVALUATION OF TEXTURE TEST OBJECTS FOR MAGNETIC RESONANCE IMAGING

A. MATERKA AND M. STRZELECKI

Institute of Electronics, Technical University of Łódź, Stefanowskiego 18, 90-924 Łódź, Poland, E-mail: materka@ck-sg.p.lodz.pl

R. LERSKI

Medical Physics Department, Ninewells Hospital and Medical School, Dundee DD1 9SY, UK, E-mail: r.a.lerski@dundee.ac.uk

L. SCHAD

Deutsches Krebsforschungszentrum Abt. Radiologie, Im Neuenheimer Feld 280, D-69120 Heidelberg, Germany, E-mail: l.schad@dkfz-heidelberg.de

Texture analysis of test object (phantom) images for standardization of *in vivo* magnetic resonance imaging is considered in this paper. The test objects are made of reticulated foam embedded in agarose gel. Different porosity foam materials are used to manufacture the phantoms. Both optical and MR images are analyzed, split into classes differing by the foam pore size. To characterize the image texture, a number of its first- and second-order statistical features is computed. The usefulness of the features to object class discrimination is evaluated using the ratio F of between-classes variance to within-classes variance, and multidimensional analysis of variance. The effect of noise and MR slice thickness on F is investigated.

1 Introduction

Studies have been carried out [4] to investigate whether texture measurements are transportable between magnetic resonance centers and to make firm conclusions as to the machine settings and sequence selection required. Development of quantitative methods of texture analysis of magnetic resonance images is now the subject of COST B11 European Community project scheduled for the years 1998-2002. The aim of this project is to develop methods, which would allow reliable discrimination of different kinds of tissue in MR images, independent of scanner type and place of its installation. There is an expectation that the texture analysis technique will contribute to more objective and repeatable medical diagnosis.

2 Test object images

The use of texture analysis in magnetic resonance imaging requires the availability of texture test objects (phantoms) for use in standardization of *in vivo* measurements. Four physical phantoms were manufactured in Medical Physics Department, University of Dundee, Scotland. They are in the form of glass tubes filled with different-porosity reticulated foam. The foam is stuffed with agarose gel that possesses a relatively long value of magnetic resonance T2 response [5]. The tubes were sealed properly to prevent the water included in the gel from evaporation. A series of magnetic resonance images of the phantoms were recorded using a Siemens Magnetom 1.5-Tesla scanner at the German Research Cancer Center, Heidelberg, Germany. The images represent cross-sections of the foam-filled tubes, taken at different field of view (100 mm×100 mm and 200 mm×200 mm), constant number of image pixels (256×256), different values of slice thickness (2 mm and 4 mm) – all acquired at 5 different positions along the tube axis. As a result, 4 different texture classes were obtained with five samples in each class, in this initial study. Example of the MR textured images is presented in Figure 1. Phantom images are analyzed in the current stage of investigation, before *in vivo* experiments on tissue texture analysis – planned for the future – are carried on.

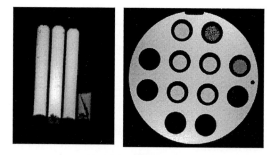

Figure 1. Test tubes (a), magnetic resonance image of the phantom cross-sections (b)

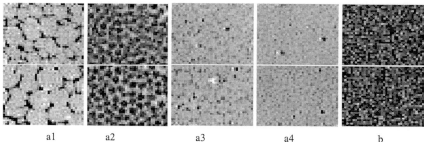

a1   a2   a3   a4   b

Figure 2. Typical ROIs from MR phantom images: a1 – coarse foam; a2 – glass bead; a3 – medium foam; a4 – smooth foam; b – background noise. Slice thickness: upper row – 4 mm, lower row – 2 mm.

Independently, optical images of the reticulated foam materials were digitally recorded, for comparison with MR images. They contain scans of cross-section of two different-porosity foams. Figure 2 shows the obtained 8-bit images of size 175x175 pixels. From each optical image, 48 non-overlapping samples of size 23x23 pixels were taken, resulting in 2 texture classes, each of 48 samples.

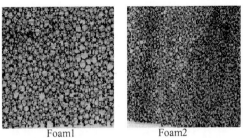

Foam1   Foam2

Figure 2. Optical images of reticulated foam materials:
Foam1 – coarse foam, Foam2 – medium pore size.

3　Results and discussion

A number of subroutines in Matlab and a specialized MS Windows application program MaZda [3] were written to compute a variety of texture features (parameters), including first-order (histogram-based), second-order (computed from co-occurrence and run-length matrices) [1], gradient, and autoregressive (AR) model-based features [2]. The programs were applied to the recorded MR and optical images to compute texture features and thus characterize texture properties. In the case of MR images, the effect of noise was taken into account by adding Gaussian noise of specified standard deviation to image samples and then computing the features. To investigate any feature ability to discriminate between different pore-size textures, the following F coefficient was used:

$$F = \frac{D}{V}$$

that represents the ratio of between-classes feature variance D to within-classes feature variance V [6].

For each sample (region of interest – ROI) of an optical image, the following 254 features were calculated:

- 9 histogram-based (mean, variance, skewness, kurtosis and five histogram percentiles for 1%, 10%, 50%, 90%, and 99%: #1 – #9); H,
- 5 gradient-based features (absolute gradient mean, variance, skewness, kurtosis, and percentage of non-zero gradients: #10 – #14); GR,
- 20 run-length matrix-based features (short run emphasis inverse moment, long run emphasis moment, gray level nonuniformity, run length nonuniformity and

fraction of image in runs, separately for horizontal, vertical, 45° and 135° directions: #15 – #34); LB,

- 220 co-occurrence matrix based features (11 features defined in [1] calculated for matrices constructed for five distances between image pixels (d=1, 2, 3, 4 and 5), and for the four directions as in the case of RL features: #35 – #254; CO.

Except for the histogram-based features, each ROI image was quantized to 64 gray levels (6-bit word-length) prior to computation of the texture parameters.

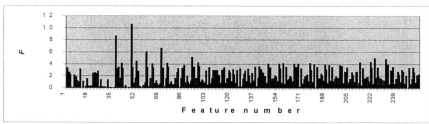

Figure 3. F coefficient for H, GR, RL and CO features (no ROI normalization).

For each of the above-mentioned features, F coefficient was computed to express the possibility to separate the two foam classes based on a given feature. As presented in Figure 3, for raw images, i.e. with no image normalization within ROIs, only 4 features from the whole set (#37, #48, #59, and #70) represent relatively high value of F coefficient (e.g. $F \geq 6.0$). They are correlation coefficients calculated for the co-occurrence matrix determined at $d = 1$, for the four main directions. Other features possess lower F values, which means that they are not very useful to make distinction between the two classes of the foam texture (Table 1).

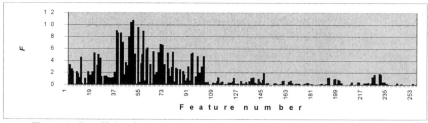

Figure 4. F coefficient for H, GR, RL and CO features ('±3 sigma' ROI normalization).

To investigate whether image normalization has an influence on feature ability to allow discrimination between the image classes, two normalization schemes were considered. For both schemes, the image histogram was first computed within each ROI. Then, the image mean μ and standard deviation σ were found. For the '±3 sigma' scheme, the image intensity levels were limited to the range from a minimum of $f_{min}=\mu-3\sigma$ to a maximum of $f_{max}=\mu+3\sigma$. The intensity range ($f_{max}-f_{min}$) was then quantized using 6-bit word-length prior to computation of GR, RL and CO parameters. On the other hand, for the '1% – 99%' scheme, the values of f_{min} and f_{max} were determined as corresponding to, respectively, 1% and 99% of cumulative image histogram within ROI.

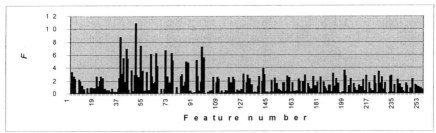

Figure 5. F coefficient for H, GR, RL and CO features ('1%–99%' ROI normalization).

The F coefficient distribution among the different texture features, obtained for the '±3 sigma' and '1%–99%' normalization schemes is illustrated in Fig. 4 and Fig. 5, respectively. Indeed, for '±3 sigma' scheme, the number of features that have high F ($F \geq 6.0$) increased significantly to 12. An intermediate number of 9 such features was obtained for '1%–99%' scheme. Numerical results of this experiment are presented in Table 1.

Table 1. F coefficient for different normalization schemes (numbers in bold: $F>6$).

No.	Feature definition	Feature number	F, no normalization	F '±3 sigma'	F '1%–99%'
1	(1,0) Contrast	36	0.2	**9.0**	2.4
2	(1,0) Correlation	37	**8.7**	**8.6**	**8.8**
3	(1,0) Inverse Differential Moment	39	3.5	**8.7**	5.5
4	(1,0) Sum Variance	41	4.1	**7.1**	**7.0**
5	(1,0) Differential Entropy	45	0.0	**8.0**	3.6
6	(0,1) Contrast	47	0.1	**10.4**	2.9
7	(0,1) Correlation	48	**10.6**	**10.7**	**10.9**
8	(0,1) Sum Variance	52	4.4	**9.6**	**7.5**
9	(0,1) Differential Entropy	56	0.1	**9.0**	3.4
10	(1,1) Correlation	59	**6.1**	**6.2**	**6.1**
11	(1,1) Sum Variance	63	4.0	5.6	**6.3**
12	(1,-1) Contrast	69	0.8	**6.7**	0.8
13	(1,-1) Correlation	70	**6.6**	**6.6**	**6.7**
14	(1,-1) Sum Variance	74	4.1	5.3	**6.3**
15	(0,2) Sum Variance	96	4.2	4.7	**7.3**

It is evident that the number of useful features depends significantly on image normalization. To explain this effect, one should refer to image properties as seen in

Figure 2. Namely, the images investigated, especially 'Foam2', show some nonuniformity of their local mean and variance. It can be found that relative standard deviation σ_μ of image mean μ, computed over 48 ROIs, is equal to $\sigma_\mu/\mu=12.2\%$ for 'Foam1' and as much as $\sigma_\mu/\mu=24.2\%$ for 'Foam2'. Similarly, the corresponding ratios related to image variance are equal to 15.8% for 'Foam1' and 29.1% for 'Foam2'. At the same time, F coefficient for image mean μ is equal to 1.6 and that for image variance σ^2 equals to 3.4. One can then expect that if there exist texture features, which possess high correlation to μ and σ^2, and image is not normalized, then such features will demonstrate non-zero values of F even if they do not carry any information about texture properties other than μ and σ^2. Such features will be redundant in a given application. Moreover, high correlation to μ and σ^2 may mask a feature ability to discriminate the texture classes.

To find out whether there are indeed features highly correlated to μ and σ^2 (within the feature set under consideration) two numerical experiments were carried out – one with modified image mean value, and the other with a modified variance. For each texture feature, the ratio of its value after mean (variance) modification to the value before modification was calculated, as presented in Figure 6.

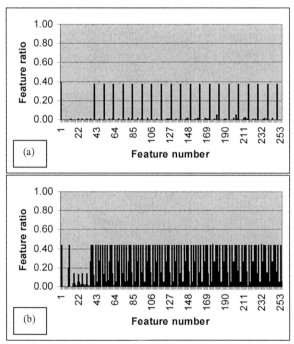

Figure 6. The effect of image mean (a) and variance (b) on texture features.

The increase in image mean corresponding to Figure 6a is equal to 0.39 of its non-modified value. Similar increase (0.37) is observed for the CO Sum Average features, regardless of the distance d and direction used for CO matrix computation. These features are represented by 20 respective bars in Figure 6a, numbered as 40, 51, ..., 249. The GR (#10-#14) and RL (#15-#34) features did not depend on μ, as can be expected. The histogram percentile features (#5 - #9) were set to zero to neglect the effect of slight intensity clipping due to the modifications.

Figure 6b indicates that many more features depend on σ^2 (#2) compared to μ. The increase in σ^2 shown in this Figure equals to 0.44. The same increase is observed for gradient variance (#11). The gradient mean is increased by a factor of 0.2 (#10). As far as RL features are concerned, the increase of 0.14 is measured for the so-called Run Length Nonuniformity [1], regardless of the direction (#16, #21, #26, and #31). Most of the CO-derived features demonstrate dependence on σ^2. The same increase of 0.44 is obtained for CO Contrast (#36), CO Sum of Squares (#38), CO Sum Variance (#41) and CO Difference Variance (#44). The CO Angular Second Moment (#35) increased by 0.27, and the CO Inverse Difference Moment (#39) changed by a factor of 0.12. Only CO Correlation (#37) is independent of image variance. The CO features numbered from #35 to #45 correspond to all pairs of image points that are a vector $(1,0)$ apart from each other. The whole pattern of CO feature dependence on σ^2 repeats in Figure 6b with a period of 11, until the features obtained for the displacement vector $(5,-5)$ that are numbered from #244 to #254.

More detailed analysis shows that standard deviation of the mean of 'Foam1' equals to 7.8, 0.2, and 4.5, respectively for 'no normalization', '±3 sigma', and '1%-99%' schemes. The corresponding figures for 'Foam2' are equal to 11.3, 0.2, and 3.5. Thus '±3 sigma' scheme provides the best stabilization of the image mean value within the $(f_{max}-f_{min})$ window. This results in the highest number of the discriminative features (Fig. 4), thanks to elimination of the effect of their correlation to mean and variance [$\mu=0$ and σ^2 is constant relative the $(f_{max}-f_{min})$ intensity range for the '±3 sigma' normalization scheme]. Table 1 indicates that CO Correlation does not indeed depend on image normalization.

To extend the set of texture features beyond those discussed so far, a small-neighborhood AR model parameters θ_1, θ_2, θ_3, θ_4, and σ_{ar} were used [2]:

$$f_s = \sum_{r \in N_s} \theta_r f_r + e_s$$

where f_s is image intensity at site s, e_s denotes an i.i.d. driving noise of standard deviation σ_{ar}, θ_i, $i=1,...,4$ represent selected pixel-to-pixel relationship, σ_{ar} is the noise standard deviation and N_s is a neighborhood of s. The image sample mean and variance were both normalized to, respectively, 0 and 1 in the case of AR model identification. The F values obtained for AR parameters are presented in Figure 7b. In this case, three AR parameters have relatively high F values: θ_1, θ_3, and σ_{ar}. They can be used for foam textures discrimination. This is diagrammed in Figure 7c. As can be observed, the σ_{ar} feature alone is sufficient to discriminate the two optical textures.

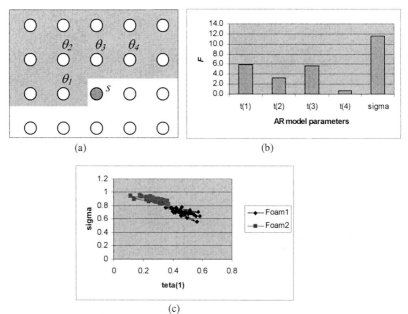

(a)

(b)

(c)

Figure 7. AR model neighborhood (a), F coefficient for AR model parameters (b), scatter-plot of two AR model features (c) – optical foam images.

In this preliminary study, the number of MR image samples for each of the 5 texture classes illustrated in Fig. 1 was limited to 5 only (25 images for each slice thickness were available, total of 50 images in the whole experiment). This eliminates the possibility of training e.g. a neural-network classifier, without its overtraining. Such attempts have then been postponed for future study, when more MR image samples are collected. Nevertheless, with the material at hand, it was still possible to draw some consistent conclusions with regard to the effects of slice thickness and noise on the class separability measure. The above-defined 5-parameter AR model was used to characterize the measured MR images of the test objects.

Figure 8 shows the F coefficient as a function of noise standard deviation (added to the images shown in Fig. 1) – calculated for all, five AR model parameters of MR images. As can be observed, discrimination ability decreases with increasing noise standard deviation. Also, the discrimination measure is higher in the case of 2-mm slice images, because for thinner slice, pores located in deeper layers distort the original (cross-sectional) texture structure to a lower extent. The effect of this distortion is especially visible in Figure 1, where images from upper and lower image rows can compare to each other.

It follows from the numerical experiments that it is possible to classify the 5 MR texture classes with no error, based on the small-neighborhood AR model parameters. However, one should remember that the sample size is very small in this study and further justification of the possibility is necessary, based on more extensive experimental material. The discrimination measure, as illustrated in Figure 8, seems to show monotonous deterioration with both slice thickness and noise. Both of these parameters of the magnetic resonance imaging process have the effect on the time of MR image measurement, and thus its cost and independence of patient body movement. It is expected that some guidelines can be formulated in future as to the time required to ensure image quality that would guarantee texture classification with a prescribed permissible error.

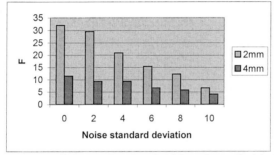

Figure 8. F coefficient as a function of additive noise standard deviation for AR model parameters (MR images).

4 Conclusions

An attempt has been made to evaluate the effectiveness of statistical parameters as texture features to discriminate between different test objects for magnetic resonance imaging. Surprisingly, only a few among more than 200 popular features are useful to distinguish the otherwise quite distinct (at least for humans) textures. This indicates the need for carrying on research work on better understanding of texture properties and for finding new feature definitions that would provide means for firm discrimination of different images of biological origin. The significance of image normalization prior to texture parameter computation has been demonstrated. This early study shows usefulness of AR model parameters for both MR and optical texture discrimination. For the future, the following investigations are planned:

- consideration of new texture features (e.g. wavelet and mathematical morphology based features),
- comprehensive analysis of noise influence on classification accuracy and selection of features that would be weakly dependent on noise,

- further development of MaZda software used for feature calculation,
- development of feature selection methods for MR texture test objects,
- extending the results to texture classification of biological tissue.

5 Acknowledgment

This work was performed within the framework of COST B11 European project. It was supported in part by British-Polish Joint Research Programme.

References

1. Haralick R., Shanmugam K. and Dinstein I., Textural features for image classification, *IEEE Trans. Systems Man Cybernetics*, **3**, 6 (1973) pp. 610-621.
2. Hu Y. and Dennis T., Textured image segmentation by context enhanced clustering, *IEE Proc.-Visual Image and Signal Processing*, **141**, 6 (1994) pp. 413-421.
3. Internet (1999) http://phase.pki.uib.no/~costb11/.
4. Lerski R., Straughan K., Schad L., Boyce D., Bluml S. and Zuna I., MR image texture analysis – an approach to tissue characterization, *Magnetic Resonance Imaging* **11** (1993) pp. 873-887.
5. Lerski R. and Schad L., The use of reticulated foam in texture test objects for magnetic resonance imaging, *Magnetic Resonance Imaging* **16**, 9 (1998) pp. 1139-1144.
6. Shürmann J., *Pattern Classification* (John Wiley and Sons, New York, 1996).

APPLYING TEXTURE ANALYSIS TO INDUSTRIAL INSPECTION

O. SILVÉN

Machine Vision and Media Processing Unit, Infotech Oulu and Department of Electrical Engineering, P.O. B. 4500, FIN-90014 University of Oulu, Finland
Email: olli.silven@ee.oulu.fi

Despite the obvious needs of applications, texture analysis is a rare method in automated visual inspection outside textile industry. Most textures in the real world are non-uniform, the inspection speed requirements extreme and very difficult to satisfy at a reasonable cost using textbook methods. Furthermore, the costs of retraining the systems tend to exceed any acceptable level. This paper gives a brief overview of the problem space of applying texture analysis for industrial inspection, presenting some solutions proposed and their prerequisites.

1 Introduction

There are many potential areas of application for texture analysis in industry [1-4], but only a limited number of examples of successful exploitation of texture in inspection exist. A major problem is that textures in the real world are often non-uniform, due to changes in orientation, scale or other visual appearance. In addition, the degree of computational complexity of many of the proposed texture measures is very high. Before committing effort into selecting, developing and using texture techniques in an application, it is necessary to thoroughly understand its requirements and characteristics.

Textured materials may have defects that should be detected and identified as in crack inspection of concrete or stone slabs, or the quality characteristics of the surface should be measured as in granulometry. In many applications both objectives must be pursued simultaneously, as is regularly the case with wood, steel and textile inspection. Because these and most natural and manufactured surfaces are textured, one would expect this characteristic to be reflected by the methodological solutions used in practical automatic visual inspection systems.

However, only a few examples of successful explicit exploitation of texture techniques in industrial inspection exist, while most systems, including many wood inspection devices, attempt to cancel out or disregard the presence of texture, trying to transform the problems solvable with other detection and analysis methods, e.g., as done by Dinstein *et al.* [5]. This is understandable against the high costs of texture inspection, and the fact that often the defects of interest are not textured, but embedded in it like cracks. Furthermore, as is the case with wood, the texture of the sound material may vary greatly, causing training problems for texture inspection algorithms.

The inspection of textured surfaces is regularly treated more as a classification and less as a segmentation task, simply because the focus is on measuring the characteristics of regions and comparing them to prior trained samples. Actual working texture based industrial inspection solutions are available mostly for homogeneous periodic textures, such as on wallpaper and fabric, where the patterns normally exhibit only minimal variation, making defect detection a two category classification problem. Natural textures are more or less random with large non-anomalous deviations, as anyone can testify by taking a look at a wood surface, resulting in the need to add features just to capture the range of normal variation, not to mention of the detection and identification of defects.

Defect detection may require continuous adaptation or adjustment of features and methods based on the background characteristics, possibly resulting in a complex multicategory classification task already at the first step of inspection. Solutions providing adaptability have been proposed, among others, by Dewaele *et al.* [6] and Chetverikov [7]. Proprietary adaptation schemes are regularly used in commercial inspection systems.

In most industrial applications inspection systems must process 10-40 Mpixels/s per camera, thus requiring dedicated hardware for at least part of the system, so the calculation of each new texture feature can be a significant expense that should be avoided. Therefore, the system developers try to select a few powerful straightforwardly implementable features and tune them precisely for the application problem. A prototypical solution depicted in Figure 1 uses a bank of filters or texture transforms characterising the texture and also defect primitives, each transform producing a feature image that is used in either pixel-by-pixel or window based classification of the original image data.

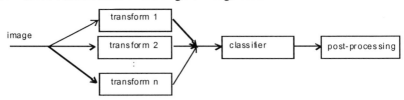

Figure 1. Typical methodological architecture of texture based inspection systems.

The dimensions of the filters used in applications have ranged up-to 63 x 63 for pixel classification [8], while most implementors rely on 3 x 3 Laws' masks [9] or other convolution filters in classification of partially overlapping or non-overlapping windows, e.g., based on means and variances of texture measures

The developments in feature distribution based classification [10,4] of texture will have a major simplifying impact on future systems, as the techniques have recently matured to the brink of real applicability. The improved efficiency in using the texture measures cuts the number of features needed in an application, enables classifying small regions, and potentially reduces training effort by relieving the dimensionality problem of classification. Nevertheless, many applications will always demand dedicated techniques for the detection of their vital defects.

2   Inspection System Training

Regardless of the feature analysis methodology, the effort needed for training an inspection system to detect and identify defects from sound background remains a key cost driver for system deployment and use. As texture inspection methods are notoriously fragile with respect to resolution, a minor change between the distance of the camera to the target may result in a retraining need. This need may also arise from normal variations between product batches.

Typically, training done in laboratory turns out to be useless after an inspection system has been installed on-line. Furthermore, on-line training performed by production personnel tends to concentrate on teaching in 'near-misses' and 'near-hits' rather than representative defects and background, so non-parametric classifiers should be favored.

Figure 2 shows two basic approaches to training defect detection: pixel-based training (2b) assumes that a human operator is able to correctly pinpoint pixels belonging to defects in the image and pixels that are from sound background. In region-based training (2c) the operator roughly labels regions that contain a defect or defects, but may also have a substantial portion of sound background, while the non-labeled regions are assumed sound.

We advocate the latter approach (2c), because it is less laborious, and because it is difficult for a human to precisely determine the boundaries of defects. It should be noticed that pixel based training disregards the transition region to defect, the characteristics of which may have high importance. For instance, the grain around a suspected defect in a lumber board helps in discriminating frequent stray bark particles from minor knots

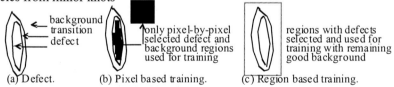

(a) Defect.   (b) Pixel based training.   (c) Region based training.

Figure 2. Alternatives for training defect detection methods.

As a practical case, it is worth considering lumber inspection in which the detection and classification of knots is essential. From Figure 3 that depicts a sound knot in a pine board we see the gradual transition from non-uniformly textured background. The great variations of the background coupled with the varying appearances of the defects clearly result in a very demanding training problem.

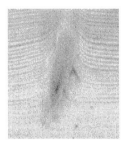

Figure 3. Typical sound leaf knot in a pine board.

3 Detection of Defects from Texture

The detection and segmentation of 'sufficiently' large defects in texture images can be performed reliably with pure texture measures both for periodic and random textures using proposed texture measures [11]. But because texture is a statistical concept, texture measures are good only for regions that have the minimum size that allows the definition of features [7].

Unfortunately, many defects are small local imperfections rather than 'real' texture defects such as knots with exactly the color of defectless background in wood. The detection of minor flaws from the background requires application specific knowledge. In addition, segmentation may be required for measuring the defects and determining their characteristics. Figure 4 presents a categorization of defects on textured surfaces.

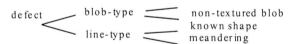

Figure 4. Categories of defects on textured surfaces.

3.1 Defect blob detection

The relative sizes of the minimum detectable defect patches for various features and textures can be roughly concluded from the boundaries in texture segmentation results given in literature: The lower the error, the smaller the defects that can be detected using that family of features. With a small patch size even most of the local texture imperfection can be detected, reducing, if not eliminating the need for application specific detection solutions for purposes such as the locating non-textured blobs from the background.

In practice, choosing the patch size for an application depends on the desired balance between false alarm and error escape rates. A smaller patch size increases the number of misdetections from normal variations, while using larger patches may contribute to detection failures. Normally all detections are subjected to further scrutiny, so in the end the patch size is defined by the general purpose computational resources available for detailed analysis.

The minimum patch size is smallest for periodic textures such as in textiles that must be inspected for both large and small weaving flaws that are generally multiplies of the mesh size. In textile inspection, Ade *et al.* [12] found that using an imaging resolution of three pixels per mesh width and averaged outputs of 3 x 3 to 5 x 5 pixel filters, derived via Karhunen-Loeve expansion of the spatial covariance matrix, the diameter of the minimum patch is around 15 pixels. The smallest detected defects in [12] appear to be around 10% of the patch area. Neubauer [13], using approximately the same imaging resolution, exploited three 5 x 5 FIR-filters and performed classification using histograms of features calculated from 10 x 10 pixel regions, achieving 1.6% false alarm and 9.3% escape rates.

The tests with LBP/C method for quasi-periodic textures performed by Ojala [14] with 16 x 16 pixel patch size and distribution classification detected 100% of the cases where more than about 25% of the block area did not belong to the same category. With natural textures the average detection threshold of other categories increased to around 35%.

3.2   Crack detection

It is evident that the inspection accuracy may significantly benefit from dedicated methods for detecting small defects. Crack or scratch detection is undoubtedly the most common defect for which specific techniques have been included in visual surface inspection systems.

The relative difficulty of detecting cracks depends on whether their shape and typical orientation is known a priori, whether they start from the edge of the object, and on whether the texture is periodic or random. A key problem is the typically very small transverse dimensions and poor contrast of cracks: the human visual system may easily detect them, but they may actually consist of 'chains' of nonadjacent single pixels in the image. In the worst case, the surface is randomly textured and the cracks may meander freely, starting and ending anywhere, leaving few application specific constraints that could be exploited.

The detection of cracks having a known shape is often straightforward applying Hough-transform or RANSAC to edge detected or high-pass filtered versions of the image. For instance, Gerhardt *et al.* [15] used Hough transform for detecting wrinkles in sandpaper in this manner.

With meandering cracks, the problem of discriminating them from other high frequency components in the image is very difficult. If the texture is periodic or quasi-periodic, texture measures characterizing the background may be powerful enough for detecting their presence. An alternative, a rather unusual simple method for defect detection from periodic patterns, based on a model of human preattentive visual detection of pattern anomalies, has been proposed by Brecher [16]. Detection is performed by comparing local and global first order density statistics of contrast or edge orientation.

Song *et al.* [17] have presented a trainable technique based on a pseudo-Wigner model for detecting cracks from periodic and random textures. The motivation behind selecting the technique is the better cojoint spatial and spatial frequency resolution offered by the Wigner distribution when compared to Gabor, difference-of-Gaussians and spectrogram approaches: this is an important factor due to the localness of cracks. The technique is trained with defectless images. During inspection it produces probabilistic distance images that are then postprocessed using rough assumptions on the shape of the cracks in the application.

4   Application Cases

Before committing effort into selecting, developing and using texture techniques in an application, it is necessary to thoroughly understand its requirements and characteristics. The developer should consider at least the following questions:

- Is the surface periodically, randomly, or only weakly textured? Strongly periodic textures can be efficiently characterized using linear filtering techniques that are also relatively cheap to implement with off-the-shelf hardware. For random textures LBP/C and gray level difference features with distribution based classification [10] are computationally attractive and rank among the very best. With weakly textured surfaces, plain gray-level and color distribution based classification may work very well [18].
- Are any of the properties of the defects known? In particular, are there any defects that cannot be discriminated from the background by their color or intensity? Due to their cost texture methods should usually be the last ones to be thrown in. They are generally much better in characterizing surfaces than in detecting anomalies. Thus, whenever feasible, application specific non-texture method solutions may be justified for detection, while texture measures may be powerful in eliminating false alarms and recognizing the defects.

The following application cases, particle size determination, carpet wear assessment and leather inspection are demonstrations of analysis of random and quasi-periodic textures, and defect detection from random textures, respectively.

4.1 Case 1: determination of particle size distribution

On-line measurement of the size distribution of granular materials, e.g., coke, minerals, pellets, etc., is a common problem in process industry, where knowledge of the mean particle size and shape of the distribution are used for control. The traditional particle size distribution measurement instruments, such as sieves, are suitable for off-line use in laboratory. The off-the-shelf machine vision systems developed for this purpose are based on blob analysis and require mechanical set-ups for separating the particles from each other. Separation is often necessary, because smaller particles may fall to the spaces between the bigger ones and are no longer visible, so the particle size distribution of the surface may not be representative. This happens if the relative size range as particle diameter is around 1.5 or larger.

Texture analysis has clear potential in granulometric applications. In principle, a measurement instrument could be trained with pictures of typical distributions, but the preparation of samples with known distributions is a laborious task, making this approach unattractive. Furthermore, the training problem is amplified by the need for frequent recalibrations, because the appearance of the material may change with time. The desired approach is to train the instrument by sieved fractions of the material, or to eliminate the need for training, as is the case with particle separation based measurements.

Rautio *et al.* [19] performed distribution measurement experiments using chrome concentrate that was sieved into 15 fractions, 37 to 500 μm, for use as training samples, and mixtures of three adjacent fractions were prepared for use as test samples. Various texture features, and distribution based and ordinary statistical classifiers were used in analysis. Figure 5 shows examples of the training material and mixtures, imaged at 7 x 7 μm resolution. The relative diameter range of particles in each mixture was 1.7 which results in only a minor "autosieving" phenomenon.

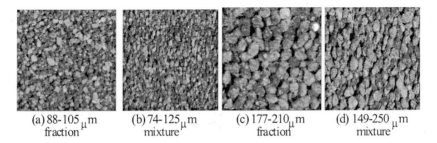

(a) 88-105 μm fraction (b) 74-125 μm mixture (c) 177-210 μm fraction (d) 149-250 μm mixture

Figure 5. Examples of sieved fractions and mixtures.

Gray level differences were found to be the best performing features with all classification schemes. Using the G metric and kNN classifier (k=3), the error of the leave-one-out test for training samples was 6%, when the gray level difference histograms with displacement 2 were used. The classification of mixture samples was performed by counting the classes of highest probability training samples, assuming that the relative counts represent the size distribution.

The measurement errors with test compositions were close to 50% for fractions below 125 μm, and around 22% for larger particle sizes. The overall error for the average size determination was 13%.

4.2   Case 2: carpet wear assessment

The assessment of appearance changes due to wear is a key factor in grading carpets. Typically, mechanical wear testers are used both during carpet development and production to produce samples that are then subjectively evaluated by panels of experts, but objective automated assessments are desired.

Siew et al. [20] performed a study to find image based measures that correlate with carpet wear. They considered and comparatively evaluated the power of statistics of spatial gray-level co-occurrence matrices, gray-level difference probability densities, gray level run-length matrices, and neighboring gray-level dependency matrices.

For experiments, four wool carpets with seemingly quasi-periodically textured appearance were selected and subjected to various durations of wear. Imaging was performed at 0.27 x 0.30 mm resolution, but at 0.54 x 0.60 mm for the coarsest texture. In the experiments the absolute percentage change in feature values with respect to the unworn control samples was computed.

It was found that while all the tested methods are promising for measuring carpet textures changes during wear, some of the features designed to measure specific characteristics work well only for certain textures. The neighboring gray-level dependency matrix based features had the best overall discrimination capabilities, followed by gray-level difference statistics, while the run-length and spatial co-occurrence methods had difficulties in assessing the wear of the finest, most randomly textured carpet.

4.3   Case 3: leather inspection

Leather hides were sorted based on their color, thickness, gray-level variations, texture and quality that is determined on the basis of the defects. For use in manufacturing shoes, belts, furniture and other leather goods, hides were selected on the basis of their characteristics and were cut into pieces of various shapes using moulds in a manner that the pieces have the desired quality, taking into account acceptable minor defects. The defects can be categorized as area faults that are local variations of gray-level or texture, line defects that are often scars or folds of skin, and point faults that are groups of spots, whose gray-levels differ from the background. The dimensions of the smallest defects that should detected are around 2 mm.

A methodology for inspecting leather hides has been investigated by Wambacq and his co-workers [21] who found that gray-level distributions for hides are symmetric even for the areas for defects, making plain histogram based detection schemes insufficient. They make a simplifying assumption that the gray values in the image are Gaussian distributed, and check whether the pixels in a 5 x 5 neighborhood are from the distribution determined for the good part of the hide using mean, variance and edginess tests. Because parts of the faults have the same characteristics as the defectless regions, the most deviating parts of the flaws are located first using stricter confidence intervals and requiring a certain number of detections in the 5 x 5 neighborhood to avoid overdetection. The reported difficulties with the methodology were mostly with very small spot and weak line faults.

5 Summary

Despite the progress in texture analysis methodology, the application of texture analysis to industrial problems is very rare. A major problem is that textures in the real world are often not uniform, due to changes in orientation, scale or other visual appearance. In addition, the degree of computational complexity of most texture measures is very high, and the methods are difficult to train properly. Recently introduced new texture measures and distribution based classification are a genuine step toward better applicability.

References

1. T.S. Newman and A.K. Jain, A survey of automated visual inspection, Comput. Vision Image Understanding 61 (1995) 231-262.
2. M. Pietikäinen and T. Ojala, Texture analysis in industrial applications, in Image Technology - Advances in Image Processing, Multimedia and Machine Vision, ed. J.L.C. Sanz, (1996) 337-359.
3. K.Y. Song, M. Petrou and J. Kittler, Texture defect detection: a review, SPIE Vol. 1708 Applications of Artificial Intelligence X: Machine Vision and Robotics, (1992), 99-106.
4. M. Pietikäinen, T. Ojala and O. Silvén, Approaches to texture-based classification, segmentation and surface inspection, in Handbook of Pattern Recognition and Computer Vision, 2nd edition, eds. C.H. Chen, L.F. Pau, P.S.P. Wang, (1999) 711-736.

5. I. Dinstein, A. Fong, L. Ni and K. Wong, Fast discrimination between homogeneous and textured regions. in Proc. 7th Int. Conf. on Pattern Recognition, Montreal, Canada, (1984), 361-363.

6. P. Dewaele, L. Van Gool, P. Wambacq and A. Oosterlinck, Texture inspection with self-adaptive convolution filters, in Proc. 9th Int. Conf. on Pattern Recognition, Rome, Italy, (1988) 56-60.

7. D. Chetverikov, Texture imperfections. Pattern Recognition Letters 6 (1987) 45-50.

8. B.K. Ersbøll and K. Conradsen, Automated grading of wood slabs: The development of a prototype system, Industrial Metrology 2 (1992) 317-342.

9. K.I. Laws, Textured image segmentation, Report 940, Image Processing Institute, Univ. of Southern California, (1980).

10. T. Ojala, M. Pietikäinen and D. Harwood, A comparative study of texture measures with classification based on feature distributions, Pattern Recogn. 29 (1996) 51-59.

11. M. Tuceryan and A.K. Jain, Texture analysis, in Handbook of Pattern Recognition and Computer Vision, 2nd edition, eds. C.H. Chen, L.F. Pau, P.S.P. Wang, (1999) 207-248.

12. F. Ade, N. Lins and M. Unser, Comparison of various filter sets for defect detection in textiles, in Proc. 7th Int. Conf. on Pattern Recognition, Montreal, Canada, (1984) 428-431.

13. C. Neubauer, Segmentation of defects in textile fabric, in Proc. 11th Int. Conf. on Pattern Recognition, Vol. I, The Hague, The Netherlands, (1992) 688-691.

14. T. Ojala and M. Pietikäinen, Unsupervised texture segmentation using feature distributions. Pattern Recognition 32, (1999) 477-486.

15. L.A. Gerhardt, R.P. Kraft, P.D. Hill and S. Neti, Automated inspection of sandpaper products and processes using image processing. SPIE Vol. 1197 Automated Inspection and High-Speed Vision Architectures III, (1989) 191-201.

16. V. Brecher, New techniques for patterned wafer inspection based on a model of human preattentive vision, SPIE Vol. 1708 Applications of Artificial Intelligence X, (1992) 452-459.

17. K.Y. Song, M. Petrou and J. Kittler, Texture crack detection, Mach. Vision Appl. 8 (1995) 63-76.

18. O. Silvén and H. Kauppinen, Recent developments in wood inspection, Int. J. Pattern Recogn. Artif. Intell. 10 (1996) 83-95.

19. H. Rautio, O. Silven and T. Ojala, Grain size measurement using distribution classification. Proc. 10th Scandinavian Conference on Image Analysis, June 9-11, Lappeenranta, Finland (1997) 1:353-359.

20. L. Siew, R. Hodgson and E. Wood, Texture measures for carpet wear assessment, IEEE Trans. Pattern Anal. Mach. Intell. 10 (1988) 92-105.

21. P. Wamback, M. Mahy, G. Noppen and A. Oosterlinck, Visual inspection in the leather industry, in Proc. IAPR Workshop on Computer Vision, Tokyo, Japan, (1988) 153-156.

AUTOMATIC DETECTION OF ERRORS ON TEXTURES USING INVARIANT GREY SCALE FEATURES AND POLYNOMIAL CLASSIFIERS

M. SCHAEL AND H. BURKHARDT

Institute for Pattern Recognition and Image Processing,
Computer Science Department, University of Freiburg,
Am Flughafen 17, D-79110 Freiburg, Germany
E-mail: {schael,burkhardt}@informatik.uni-freiburg.de

In this paper we propose two methods for the automatic detection of errors on non-stochastic textures. Both methods are based on invariant grey scale features and may be distinguished by their global or local approach, respectively. Classification of the non-linear invariant features is done by a polynomial classifier of third degree. Our test application for the evaluation of the invariant features is the error detection on textile surfaces. Experimental results based on the image database *TILDA* are presented and discussed in this contribution.

1 Introduction

Over the last decade the automatic detection of errors on textures has gained increasing importance for industrial applications. Manufacturing of high quality products needs control. In many areas of production the quality can be assessed by analyzing planar surfaces of the product under test, e.g. textiles and wood. Visual inspection by human operators is still widely used in many areas of manufacturing. One reason for the small number of automatic visual inspection systems being used is the difficulty of modelling the knowledge of the humans who currently classify the surfaces. Furthermore, the description and modelling of textures is still a great challenge [1].

Many papers develop special solutions for specific error detection tasks, e.g. the detection of flaws on woven textiles and roll goods. Campbell et al. propose a model-based clustering method which can detect flaws in woven textiles [2]. Their idea is to derive special solutions for every single problem. Concepts for the determination of product quality are proposed by Greiner et al. [3]. The product quality of roll goods is assessed using image processing techniques. A hierarchical texture analysis based on wavelet transformation is proposed there. This method makes it possible to detect different types of errors on roll goods. To increase the acceptance of automatic visual inspection systems in a wide industrial field it is necessary to develop methods which can easily be adapted to different visual inspection tasks. Developing only specific solutions for every single error detection task produces high costs which are unacceptable for the manufacturer.

In this paper we propose two methods for the detection of errors on non-stochastic textures. Due to the different position and orientation of the texture under the camera of a visual inspection system it is necessary to construct features which are invariant with respect to these transformations. Since the distance between the camera and the surface is fixed, we do not need to consider scaling. Our approaches are based on global and local invariant features. Both methods can be used for different visual inspection tasks.

This paper is organized as follows: in the next section we introduce a method for the construction of invariant grey scale features. Two approaches for global and local invariant features are derived. The third section describes the experiments and their results. A discussion of the results is given in section four. Finally a conclusion is given.

2   Construction of invariant features

Schulz-Mirbach proposed a method for the construction of invariant features for two-dimensional grey scale images by averaging over the transformation group [4,5]. Averaging over a group G can be written as

$$A[f](\mathbf{M}) := \frac{1}{|G|} \int\limits_G f(g\mathbf{M}) \, dg, \tag{1}$$

where the fraction in front of the integral is used to normalize the averaging result by the volume of the group G. The integral is also known as Haar integral. Equation (1) is also called invariant integration. For compact groups we define the volume $|\cdot|$ of a group G as $|G| := \int_G dg$. It is evident that the result is invariant to any transformation $g \in G$ if we average over all transformed patterns $g\mathbf{M}$. For compact and finite groups the existence of a complete feature set can be shown [5]. If we choose monomials as functions f, an upper number of monomials for a complete feature set can be given [5]. In general the function f can be arbitrarily chosen. Due to the fact that we want to construct invariant features for the rotation and translation in $I\!\!R^2$ (Euclidean motion) we will now focus on the Euclidean transformation group G_E. The Euclidean group can be defined by the rotation group $SO(2)$ and the translation group G_T as the Cartesian product $G_E := SO(2) \times G_T$. The translation group G_T can be parameterized by $(t_x, t_y)^T$, which defines the translation vector $\mathbf{t}$. An element of the rotation group $g \in SO(2)$ can be parameterized by a rotation angle φ. Inserting the parameterized group G_E

into eq. (1) leads to:

$$A[f](\mathbf{M}) = \frac{1}{|G|} \int\limits_{G_E} f(g\mathbf{M})\, dg = \frac{1}{2\pi N^2} \int\limits_{t_x=0}^{N} \int\limits_{t_y=0}^{N} \int\limits_{\varphi=0}^{2\pi} f(g\mathbf{M})\, d\varphi dt_x dt_y. \quad (2)$$

Given a grey scale image $\mathbf{M}$ and an element $g \in G_E$ of the group of image translations and rotations, the transformation can be expressed as

$$(g\mathbf{M})(i,j) = \mathbf{M}(k,l) \quad \text{with} \tag{3}$$

$$\begin{pmatrix} k \\ l \end{pmatrix} = \begin{pmatrix} \cos\varphi & -\sin\varphi \\ \sin\varphi & \cos\varphi \end{pmatrix} \begin{pmatrix} i \\ j \end{pmatrix} - \begin{pmatrix} t_x \\ t_y \end{pmatrix}. \tag{4}$$

All indices are understood modulo N. Figure 2 shows the straightforward approach for the evaluation of the invariant integral formula.

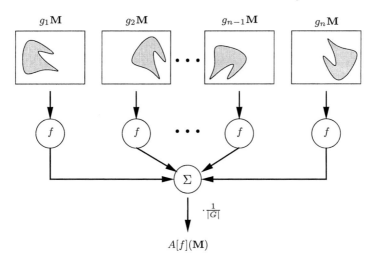

Figure 1. Evaluation of the invariant integral.

To give some intuitive insight in eq. (2) consider the following example: For the function $f(\mathbf{M}) = \mathbf{M}(0,0)\mathbf{M}(0,1)$ the group average is

$$A[f](\mathbf{M}) = \frac{1}{2\pi N^2} \int\limits_{t_x=0}^{N} \int\limits_{t_y=0}^{N} \int\limits_{\varphi=0}^{2\pi} \mathbf{M}(-t_x, -t_y)\mathbf{M}(\sin\varphi - t_x, \cos\varphi - t_y)\, d\varphi dt_x dt_y. \quad (5)$$

Let us first consider the inner integral over φ. When varying φ between 0 and 2π the second coordinate given describes a circle with radius 1 around the center $(-t_x, -t_y)$. This means we have to take the product between the center value and points on the circle and average over all these products. The remaining integrals over t_x, t_y just mean that the center point has to be varied covering the whole image. Because of the discrete image grid in practice the integrals are replaced by sums, choosing only the image grid points as centres and varying the angle in discrete steps applying bilinear interpolation for pixels that do not coincide with the image grid. For functions f of local support the calculation can generally be separated into two steps: First for every pixel a local function is evaluated, which only depends on the grey scale values in a specific neighborhood. Then all intermediate results of the local computations are summed up. The complexity is therefore linear in the image size. This alternative strategy for the evaluation of the integration is illustrated in figure 2.

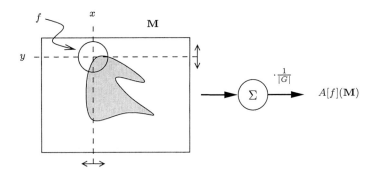

Figure 2. Alternative evaluation of the invariant integral with two step strategy.

In eq. (2) the formula for the construction of global invariant features is given. We will now derive local features based on the intermediate results. Let us define the intermediate image $\mathbf{I}$ as the result of all local computations:

$$\mathbf{I}(k,l) = \frac{1}{2\pi} \int\limits_{\varphi=0}^{2\pi} f(\mathbf{M}[g_\varphi^{-1}\begin{pmatrix} x \\ y \end{pmatrix} + \begin{pmatrix} k \\ l \end{pmatrix}]) \, d\varphi. \qquad (6)$$

where $(k,l)^T$ denotes the pixel coordinate in the intermediate image $\mathbf{I}$ and g_φ^{-1} is the inverse rotation matrix (group element of $SO(2)$). Instead of computing the global sum after the evaluation of the local computations we estimate a histogram from the intermediate image $\mathbf{I}$. Thus, we obtain a feature distribution from the local results. The traditional histogram is too sensitive to noise because of the uncontinuous assignment of values at bin boundaries. By using weighted histograms we avoid these problems. Using weighted histograms instead of global features allows us to increase the information content of the features. This technique is successfully applied to the task of texture classification [6].

By using histogram based features we are constrained to use special metrics, e.g. χ^2 or sums-of-squared-distances, for comparison. An optimal classifier cannot be applied due to the sparse histograms. To address the problem of sparse histograms where many bins contain zero entries we use a method for the estimation of adaptive histograms [7]. The idea is to apply clustering techniques, e.g. k-means, to all pixel values of the intermediate image $\mathbf{I}$ in order to determine bin prototypes. Based on the bin prototypes we compute an adaptive histogram. Since the bin entries of the adaptive histogram are no longer sparse it is possible to use an optimal classifier. Let $\{\lambda_j\}$, $i = 1, \ldots, k$, be a set of k prototypes which are determined by applying a suitable clustering method to the intermediate image. Then the adaptive histogram $\mathbf{H}_A$ is defined by:

$$H_A(\omega) = \left| \left\{ i \in \mathbf{I} : \omega = \arg\min_j \|i - \lambda_j\| \right\} \right|. \qquad (7)$$

The prototypes of the adaptive histogram depend significantly on the chosen number of clusters k. Evaluating several number of clusters allows us to find the most suitable k. Prototypes can be obtained by the following strategy: A set of image samples $\mathcal{S}$ of the reference class (the class without any error) is given. For a monomial f the histogram of the intermediate image of each sample image $\mathbf{S} \in \mathcal{S}$ can be computed. Averaging over all histograms (the number of bins is given by the range of the pixel values) of the intermediate images leads to a median histogram. The clustering is performed based on the median histogram. The derived prototypes are used for the computation of all adaptive histograms.

Since the amount of data is large one may think a statistical classifier, e.g. Bayes, should be sufficient. But we should choose a classifier depending on the properties of our invariant features. By using monomials as kernel function f we obtain non-linear features. Thus, a Bayes classifier, e.g. for normal distributions, is not be sufficient. A classifier based on a functional approximation should be appropriate. We have decided to use a polynomial classifier of third degree for the classification task.

The method's degree of freedom is given by choosing the monomial kernel functions f appropriately. Thus, our method can be adapted by the user for a given error detection task. Since we do not know which monomial is most suitable for a given application we should use a feature selection strategy. In this contribution we will not focus on the feature selection task which concerns every pattern recognition problem. For the sake of completeness though, we give two ideas on how the features can be suitably selected: Pannekamp and Schmutz propose a method for the feature selection based on the Kullback-Leibler distance [8]. The selection of feature subsets and the evaluation of their effectiveness are realized as a sequential forward search strategy. A second approach for the feature selection is given by the usage of a polynomial classifier. Strategies for the assessment of relevant polynomial terms exist [9]. Linear dependent features can be detected and removed.

3 Experiments and results

Our test application for the validation of the presented method is the detection of errors on textile textures. We have used real texture images from our textile texture database $TILDA^a$. An extensive description of the database can be found in [10]. All images of the database have size 768×512 and a dynamic of 8 bits per pixel. We have chosen a subset of images from the database $TILDA$ for the experiments. Four different textile classes ($C1R1$, $C1R3$, $C2R2$ and $C2R3$), four error classes ($E1$-$E4$) and an error-free reference class ($E0$) were used. Clippings of size 128×128 pixels of the used textile texture images are shown in figure 3. The error classes consist of $E1$ - holes in the surface, $E2$ - spots on the surface, $E3$ - thread errors and $E4$ - objects on the surface.

---

[a]The textile texture database was developed within the framework of the working group Texture Analysis of the DFG's (Deutsche Forschungsgemeinschaft) major research program "Automatic Visual Inspection of Technical Objects". The database can be obtained on two CD-ROMs on order at the URL http://www.informatik.uni-freiburg.de/~lmb/tilda.

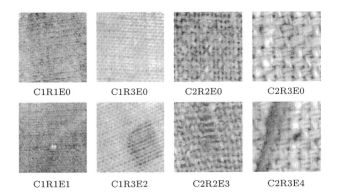

| C1R1E0 | C1R3E0 | C2R2E0 | C2R3E0 |

| C1R1E1 | C1R3E2 | C2R2E3 | C2R3E4 |

Figure 3. Clippings of textile texture images used for the experiments.

For the computation of the global and local invariant features we have used the monomials listed in table 3 as kernel function.

Table 1. Used monomials as kernel function f_i.

i	$f_i(M)$	i	$f_i(M)$
1	$M[0,0]M[5,0]$	11	$M[-5,0]M[0,5]$
2	$M[0,0]M[10,0]$	12	$M[0,5]M[0,-5]$
3	$M[0,0]M[15,0]$	13	$M[1,0]M[0,3]$
4	$M[5,0]M[10,0]$	14	$M[0,5]M[-3,0]$
5	$M[0,0]M[2,0]M[2,0]$	15	$M[-5,-3]M[3,5]$
6	$M[0,0]M[2,0]M[6,0]$	16	$M[5,3]M[1,-5]$
7	$M[2,0]M[6,0]M[6,0]$	17	$M[1,2]M[4,3]$
8	$M[2,0]M[4,0]M[6,0]$	18	$M[2,3]M[5,4]$
9	$M[-5,0]M[5,3]$	19	$M[1,0]M[0,1]$
10	$M[4,-3]M[0,5]$	20	$M[0,5]M[5,0]$

Classification is done by subsets of the features in table 3. For 2, 3 and 4 features all possible combinations of the global features were evaluated on the image set. Three different cluster sizes ($k = 3, 4$ and 5) were used for the evaluation of local features. Only one feature channel of the local features was used for classification. Training of the polynomial classifier was done by 30 of 50 samples. All remaining samples were used for the assessment of the classifier.

Table 2. Classification results of the global invariant features.

TC	n	TCR [%]	f_i	CCR[%]				
				E0	E1	E2	E3	E4
C1R1	2	70	$\{2, 15\}$	100	50	90	15	95
		55	$\{9, 11\}$	95	50	35	0	95
	3	__71__	$\{1, 11, 15\}$	100	50	85	30	90
		48	$\{2, 3, 6\}$	70	30	50	0	90
	4	69	$\{1, 3, 7, 10\}$	100	50	90	20	85
		27	$\{9, 10, 19, 20\}$	40	25	15	30	25
C1R3	2	52	$\{7, 13\}$	100	100	5	30	25
		39	$\{1, 7\}$	95	100	0	0	0
	3	__59__	$\{4, 9, 20\}$	100	100	15	40	40
		38	$\{3, 6, 9\}$	90	95	0	5	0
	4	59	$\{3, 5, 17, 20\}$	100	85	25	35	50
		32	$\{2, 6, 7, 8\}$	75	45	15	15	10
C2R2	2	55	$\{1, 11\}$	90	55	60	35	35
		35	$\{8, 9\}$	75	45	5	35	15
	3	54	$\{1, 2, 18\}$	90	65	40	25	50
		36	$\{1, 4, 5\}$	55	30	50	5	10
	4	__57__	$\{1, 6, 7, 16\}$	75	80	45	30	55
		26	$\{6, 10, 11, 16\}$	45	15	25	20	25
C2R3	2	__68__	$\{3, 15\}$	100	40	95	75	30
		46	$\{17, 20\}$	95	5	60	55	15
	3	54	$\{1, 2, 14\}$	95	0	55	80	40
		30	$\{7, 10, 11\}$	100	0	10	30	10
	4	56	$\{2, 3, 7, 14\}$	95	5	55	75	50
		24	$\{7, 9, 10, 11\}$	55	0	20	10	35

Classification results of the global and local invariant features are listed in table 2 and table 3, respectively. Each row shows the maximum and minimum classification results which could be obtained by using different kernels, feature numbers and cluster sizes. We have used the following abbreviations in both tables: TC as the textile class name (see figure 3 for a corresponding image sample). The total classification rate TCR is defined as the sum over all correct classified samples divided by the total number of classified samples for all classes. CCR denotes the class specific classification rate. In table 2 n denotes the number of used features. k denotes the number of used clusters for the construction of the adaptive histograms in table 3. The best total classification rates are underlined.

Table 3. Classification results of the local invariant features.

TC	k	TCR [%]	f_i	CCR[%]				
				E0	E1	E2	E3	E4
C1R1	3	74	{1}	85	50	100	50	85
		52	{10}	85	20	50	38	70
	4	**77**	{3}	80	70	85	50	100
		52	{11}	85	20	70	0	85
	5	72	{2}	85	70	70	50	85
		55	{10}	70	20	50	50	85
C1R3	3	58	{5}	100	100	20	70	0
		44	{4}	100	85	0	35	0
	4	74	{4}	100	100	20	100	50
		54	{10}	100	100	20	50	0
	5	**84**	{7}	100	100	70	100	50
		54	{1}	100	85	35	0	50
C2R2	3	56	{2}	100	65	50	50	15
		33	{18}	65	50	15	0	35
	4	77	{1}	85	50	65	100	85
		41	{17}	35	50	35	50	35
	5	**78**	{2}	85	85	85	50	85
		39	{17}	15	65	65	35	35
C2R3	3	66	{8}	100	35	85	85	35
		50	{14}	85	15	35	65	50
	4	**73**	{11}	100	65	85	100	15
		47	{14}	85	15	50	50	35
	5	73	{11}	100	65	85	100	15
		47	{14}	85	15	50	50	35

4   Discussion

The experimental results show an improvement of the total classification rates by using local invariant features instead of global invariant features. Furthermore, better results can be obtained by using only one kernel function. Increasing the number of global features used for the classification task does not automatically lead to better results. If we only want to discriminate two classes (texture with or without defect) both methods achieve nearly 100 %. For all three texture classes the local invariant features obtain better results. On the other hand, there are error classes which are difficult to classify, e.g. error class $E4$ of textile class $C2R3$. Bad classification results can be explained by perturbations of the textures. Due to the fact that we are using grey scale based features it must be guaranteed that perturbations like inhomogeneous illumination are minimized. All textile texture images of the database *TILDA* are perturbed by inhomogeneous illumination. It should be noted that we have only used a small set of kernel functions f. A suitable selection of monomials for a given application can only be obtained by an appropriate feature selection method. The optimization of the kernel function of a given application can be performed off-line. A suitable selection of the cluster number must be done by a selection strategy and cannot be given a priori. We have only computed three different cluster numbers. The results show that for different textile classes different cluster numbers leads to the best results. An appropriate cluster size may be optimized together with the kernel function. One explanation for the difference between the obtained results of the local and global features is the construction method. Global features are built by an averaging over all local results. This operation decimates too much information of the error image structures. Local adaptive feature histograms proved to preserve much more information than the global features.

5   Conclusion

In this paper we have proposed two methods for the automatic detection of errors on non-stochastic textures. Both methods are based on invariant grey scale features and may be distinguished by their global or local approach, respectively. The application of the global and local invariant features is not restricted to one error detection task. For both methods the underlying theory has been presented. Experiments based on real textile texture images taken from the database *TILDA* show good results. A comparison of the global and local features indicates that the local features can discriminate better between error classes.

Acknowledgements

This work was supported by the "Deutsche Forschungsgemeinschaft" (DFG).

References

1. R. M. Haralick and L. G. Shapiro. *Computer and Robot Vision*, volume 2. Addison-Wesley, 1993.
2. J. G. Campbell, C. Fraley, F. Murtagh, and A. E. Raftery. Linear flaw detection in woven textiles using model-based clustering. *Pattern Recognition Letters*, (18):1539–1548, 1997.

3. T. Greiner, C. Ansorge, and M. Kerstein. Qualitätsprüfung von Bahn-warenmaterialien. *AT-Automatisierungstechnik*, (12):566–576, 1997.

4. H. Schulz-Mirbach. Invariant features for gray scale images. In G. Sagerer, S. Posch, and F. Kummert, editors, *17. DAGM - Symposium "Mustererkennung"*, pages 1–14, Bielefeld, 1995. Reihe Informatik aktuell, Springer.

5. H. Schulz-Mirbach. *Anwendung von Invarianzprinzipien zur Merkmalgewinnung in der Mustererkennung*. PhD thesis, Technische Universität Hamburg-Harburg, February 1995. Reihe 10, Nr. 372, VDI-Verlag.

6. S. Siggelkow and H. Burkhardt. Invariant feature histograms for texture classification. In *Proceedings of the 1998 Joint Conference on Information Sciences (JCIS'98)*, Research Triangle Park, North Carolina, USA, October 1998.

7. J. M. Buhmann and J. Puzicha. Unsupervised learning for robust texture segmentation. In H. Burkhardt, editor, *Workshop on Texture Analysis 1998*. Albert-Ludwigs-Universität, Freiburg, Institut für Informatik, September 1998.

8. J. Pannekamp and M. Schmutz. Methodology for evaluation and selection of features. In H. Burkhardt, editor, *Workshop on Texture Analysis 1998*. Albert-Ludwigs-Universität, Freiburg, Institut für Informatik, September 1998.

9. J. Schürmann. *Pattern Classification: a unified view of statistical and neural approaches*. Interscience Publications. Wiley and Sons, New York, 1996.

10. H. Schulz-Mirbach. TILDA-Ein Referenzdatensatz zur Evaluierung von Sichtprüfungsverfahren für Textiloberflächen. Internal Report 4/96, Technische Informatik I, Technische Universität Hamburg-Harburg, 1996.

UNSUPERVISED SEGMENTATION OF SURFACE DEFECTS WITH SIMPLE TEXTURE MEASURES

JUKKA IIVARINEN

Helsinki University of Technology
Laboratory of Computer and Information Science
P.O. Box 5400, FIN-02015 HUT, Finland
Jukka.Iivarinen@hut.fi

In this paper a simple and fast approach to unsupervised segmentation of surface defects is described. A set of simple texture measures (the local binary pattern method) and the statistical self-organizing map are used to detect defects in surface images. Defect detection can be seen as a typical two-class segmentation problem where the desired classes are good surface and defected surface. The main idea in this paper is to train a two-class classifier only with fault-free surface samples which is an unexpected approach. The proposed defect detection is based on the following idea: an unknown sample is classified as a defect if it differs enough from the estimated distribution of fault-free samples. The statistical self-organizing map is used to estimate this distribution. Surface images are used to demonstrate the proposed procedure.

1 Introduction

Image segmentation is a fundamental problem in image analysis. The goal of image segmentation is to partition an image into a set of regions which are uniform and homogeneous. In the best case these regions will have a strong correlation with objects in the image. For example, in industrial inspection the goal of segmentation is often to separate objects from the background.

In this paper a special type of image segmentation, a two-class segmentation, is considered. A typical two-class problem is defect detection of surfaces (see a review on texture defect detection [1]) where one of the main requirements is that the defect detection algorithm should be simple, efficient, and realizable in a given hardware architecture. Texture is an important characteristic of many types of images and is hence commonly used in image segmentation, referred to as texture segmentation. Many different approaches to texture have been proposed [2,3,4,5]. Texture-based techniques have been applied in surface defect detection since the early 1980's [6,7,8,9,10,11,12]. Especially feature-based histogram techniques have been popular since they are fast to compute (or can at least be approximated with fast algorithms) and they are relatively simple methods. Still many commercial systems today [13,14,15] are based on more simple methods, in particular on gray level thresholding techniques.

In surface defect detection a classifier is typically trained with samples taken only from a fault-free surface [6,16,7]. This results in many benefits. A tedious collection of defects is not needed and appearance of new defects do not result in retraining of a classifier. Features extracted from fault-free surface samples are usually assumed to follow a multidimensional Gaussian distribution so that the decision function can be formulated. The segmentation scheme that is used in this paper does not have this restriction; the distribution can be of any shape. The statistical self-organizing map is used to estimate the distribution of fault-free surface samples [11,17].

2 The Unsupervised Segmentation Procedure

The segmentation procedure used in the experiments is done as follows. An image is scanned with a small gliding window. A feature vector is extracted from the gliding window for a center image pixel. Each image pixel is then classified as a defect or as a fault-free pixel. Two different steps are thus recognized (Fig. 1):

1. **Feature extraction**
   Calculate a set of texture features for a given image window. Collect these features into a feature vector $\mathbf{f}$.

2. **Segmentation**
   Compare $\mathbf{f}$ with the statistical SOM and find the best-matching unit c (Eq. 1 and 2). Show the minimum error e_c as the output. If $e_c > 0$, the pixel is classified as a defect. Otherwise the pixel is fault-free.

The problem can thus be stated as: *Label the center pixel of the given image window as a defect or as a fault-free pixel.*

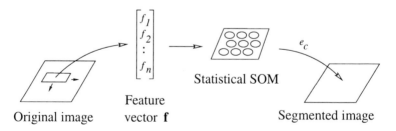

Figure 1. The proposed segmentation scheme.

2.1 The Statistical Self-Organizing Map

An extension to the original SOM algorithm, the statistical SOM, is used as a classifier [11,17]. It is a simple and fast algorithm that is used to determine if a given unknown sample belongs to a distribution of previously encountered samples. No Gaussian assumptions of the shape of the distribution have to be made; instead, the distribution can be of any shape. The basic idea in the statistical SOM is to fit a one-dimensional density function to each component plane of the Voronoi set of each map unit, and then determine a confidence interval to each one-dimensional density function.

The statistical SOM is calculated in two steps. First the SOM is trained with fault-free samples, and then a new error function is formulated to each SOM unit. The error e_i between the feature vector $\mathbf{f}$ and the statistical SOM unit i is a kind of Hamming distance,

$$e_i = \sum_{j=1}^{n} e_{ij}, \text{ where } e_{ij} = \begin{cases} 0 \text{ if } (f_j - m'_{ij})^2 \leq \left(\frac{d'_{ij}}{2}\right)^2 \\ 1 \text{ otherwise,} \end{cases} \tag{1}$$

where m'_{ij} is the jth component of a weight vector $\mathbf{m}'_i$ of a statistical SOM unit i, d'_{ij} is the jth component of a confidence interval vector $\mathbf{d}'_i$ of a statistical SOM unit i, and n is the feature space dimension. The e_i determines on how many feature planes the feature vector $\mathbf{f}$ differs from the unit i. The best-matching map unit c is now chosen to be the unit with the minimum error e_c,

$$e_c = \min_i \{e_i\}. \tag{2}$$

For details on how the the weight vectors $\mathbf{m}'_i$ and the confidence interval vectors $\mathbf{d}'_i$ are calculated, see [17].

3 Feature Extraction

Three simple measures are used for texture characterization: a local binary pattern (LBP), a simple contrast measure, and a mean value. These measures are extracted from small 3x3 image windows. The LBP and the contrast measure are defined in the following, and the mean value is simply the average of all the nine pixels in a 3x3 image window.

3.1 A Local Binary Pattern

A local binary pattern (LBP) method is a two-level version of the texture unit method [18]. It has been used successfully in metal surface inspection [9] and it performed well in a recent comparison [19]. The texture unit elements $TU_k(\mathbf{x})$, $k = 1, 2, ..., 8$, are simple functions of gray level values I around a given pixel position $\mathbf{x}$. The texture unit element $TU_k(\mathbf{x})$ is given as

$$TU_k(\mathbf{x}) = \begin{cases} 0 \text{ if } I(\mathbf{x} + \mathbf{d}_k) < I(\mathbf{x}), \\ 1 \text{ if } I(\mathbf{x} + \mathbf{d}_k) \geq I(\mathbf{x}) \end{cases} \tag{3}$$

where $\mathbf{d}_k$, $k = 1, 2, ..., 8$, are displacement vectors. They define a 3×3 neighborhood (from left to right and from top to bottom) of the center pixel $\mathbf{x}$.

The texture unit number TN is a unique number that is assigned to each different binary pattern in a 3x3 window,

$$TN(\mathbf{x}) = \sum_{k=1}^{8} TU_k(\mathbf{x}) 2^{k-1}. \tag{4}$$

For each 3x3 image window, there are $2^8 = 256$ possible texture unit numbers.

3.2 A Simple Contrast Measure

In addition to the texture unit number TN, a simple contrast measure was also proposed in [19]. It is computed after the texture unit element calculation and it is a difference of the mean gray level values of the pixels with $TU_k(\mathbf{x}) = 1$ and the pixels with $TU_k(\mathbf{x}) = 0$.

4 Experimental Setup and Results

Surface defect detection is used to test the proposed scheme. It is a typical two-class segmentation problem. Defect detection is based on the following idea: an unknown sample is classified as a defect if it differs enough from the estimated prototypes of the distribution of features extracted from fault-free samples. So only samples taken from a fault-free surface are needed in training. The statistical self-organizing map is used to estimate the distribution of fault-free samples.

The surface images were quantized to 256 gray levels. The statistical SOM had 25 units. The size of the training set was 100000 feature vectors extracted from fault-free samples taken randomly from the image in Fig. 2. It is important to have enough training data available, otherwise the density estimation cannot be done accurately.

The LBP is a gray-level invariant measure. The contrast is invariant to shifting of the gray-scale but not to scaling. In our case, these features find mainly border areas between defects and a good surface, and also even areas like holes. The mean value brings the gray-level dependency into the feature

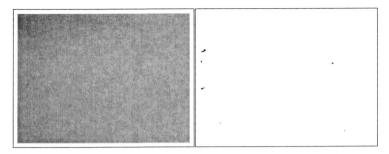

Figure 2. A surface image used for training and its segmentation with the proposed method. Defects are marked with black color.

set and fills defect areas, but also finds dark defects whose borders are smooth (the LBD and the contrast will not find these ones). The mean value is an essential feature here since many dark defects have their texture similar to a good surface; only the average gray-level value is different. Thus these defects cannot be found only with gray-level invariant texture measures. On the other hand, there are other defects that cannot be found with pure gray-level thresholding. So in this case there is a need for both the gray-level invariant measures and the gray-level dependent measures.

In Fig. 2 is the surface image that was used in training and its segmentation. As expected, only few pixels are classified as a defect. Three defect images (that were not used in training) with their segmentations are shown in Fig. 3. The whole test set consisted of 87 defect images. The morphological closing operation has been applied to all segmentations to close small gaps between found defects. The first image has some dark spots, the second image has a large hole with some dark and light areas around it, and the third image has a few holes with some weak areas around them. All defects are found nicely and accurately. There are only few misclassifications due to slight formation errors and noise. It is important for a defect detection algorithm that no good surface is classified as a defect. This is more important than to detect every weak defect.

We have previously used the co-occurrence matrix features, namely energy, contrast, and mean, in feature extraction [11,17]. The results obtained with them and with the LBP features have no critical difference in performances. The differences are found in computational requirements where the LBP features are better in several aspects: smaller image windows can be used, less memory is required, and the features are faster to compute.

5 Conclusions

The results of experiments with surface images are encouraging. The proposed scheme offers several advantages over the traditional gray-level thresholding schemes. It is general in the sense that it can be applied to defect detection of different types of surfaces. The characteristics of a fault-free surface are learned automatically from samples which results in a fast and easy learning of new surfaces. The texture features are simple ones and they are calculated from small 3x3 image windows which makes them a promising approach when considering real-time implementations.

Acknowledgements

The author wishes to thank the ABB Industry Oy and the Technology Development Centre of Finland for financial support (TEKES's grant 4172/95).

References

1. K. Y. Song, M. Petrou, and J. Kittler. Texture defect detection: A review. In *Applications of Artificial Intelligence X: Machine Vision and Robotics*, Proc. SPIE 1708, pp. 99–106, 1992.
2. R. M. Haralick. Statistical and structural approaches to texture. *Proceedings of the IEEE*, 67(5):786–804, May 1979.
3. H. Wechsler. Texture analysis – a survey. *Signal Processing*, 2(3):271–282, July 1980.
4. L. Van Gool, P. Dewaele, and A. Oosterlinck. Texture analysis anno 1983. *Computer Vision, Graphics and Image Processing*, 29(3):336–357, March 1983.
5. M. Tuceryan and A. K. Jain. Texture analysis. In *Handbook of Pattern Recognition and Computer Vision*, pp. 235–276. World Scientific, Singapore, 1993.
6. M. Unser and F. Ade. Feature extraction and decision procedure for automated inspection of textured materials. *Pattern Recognition Letters*, 2(3):185–191, March 1984.
7. F. S. Cohen, Z. Fan, and S. Attali. Automated inspection of textile fabrics using textural models. *IEEE Transactions on Pattern Analysis and Machine Intelligence*, 13(8):803–808, August 1991.
8. C. Neubauer. Segmentation of defects in textile fabric. In *Proceedings of the 11th IAPR International Conference on Pattern Recognition*, vol. I, pp. 688–691, The Hague, The Netherlands, August 30–September 3 1992.

9. M. Pietikäinen, T. Ojala, J. Nisula, and J. Heikkinen. Experiments with two industrial problems using texture classification based on feature distributions. In *Intelligent Robots and Computer Vision XIII: 3D Vision, Product Inspection and Active Vision*, Proc. SPIE 2354, pp. 197–204, 1994.

10. D. Brzakovic and N. Vujovic. Designing a defect classification system: A case study. *Pattern Recognition*, 29(8):1401–1419, 1996.

11. J. Iivarinen, J. Rauhamaa, and A. Visa. Unsupervised segmentation of surface defects. In *Proceedings of the 13th International Conference on Pattern Recognition*, vol. IV, pp. 356–360, Wien, Austria, August 25–30 1996.

12. A. Meier and U. Priber. On-line surface inspection with fuzzy-asic modules. In *5th European Congress on Intelligent Techniques and Soft Computing*, vol. 3, pp. 2474–2479, Aachen, Germany, September 8–11 1997.

13. J. C. Badger. An automatic web inspection system with advanced defect detection and classification capabilities. In *Proceedings of 1992 Nonwovens Conference*, pp. 69–80, Marco Island, Florida, May 10–14 1992.

14. J. E. Graf, S. T. Enright, and S. I. Shapiro. Automated web inspection ensures highest quality nonwovens. *Tappi Journal*, 78(9):135–138, 1995.

15. L. Mäkelin, J. Moisio, and J. Järvinen. From hole detection to image processing and information technology. In *Proceedings of 50th Appita Annual General Conference*, vol. 1, pp. 817–822, 1996.

16. P. Dewaele, L. Van Gool, P. Wambacq, and A. Oosterlinck. Texture inspection with self-adaptive convolution filters. In *Proceedings of the 9th International Conference on Pattern Recognition*, vol. 1, pp. 56–60, Rome, Italy, November 14–17 1988.

17. J. Iivarinen and A. Visa. Unsupervised image segmentation with the self-organizing map and statistical methods. In *Intelligent Robots and Computer Vision XVII: Algorithms, Techniques, and Active Vision*, Proc. SPIE 3522, pp. 516–526, 1998.

18. D.-C. He and L. Wang. Texture features based on texture spectrum. *Pattern Recognition*, 24(5):391–399, 1991.

19. T. Ojala, M. Pietikäinen, and D. Harwood. A comparative study of texture measures with classification based on feature distributions. *Pattern Recognition*, 29(1):51–59, January 1996.

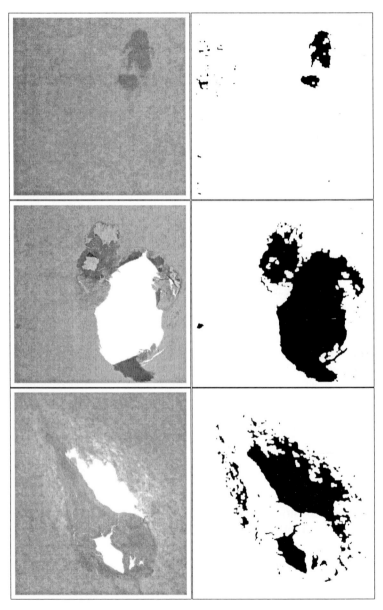

Figure 3. Surface images and their segmentations with the proposed method. Defects are marked with black color.

ANGULAR TEXTURE DISCRIMINATION OF WOODGRAIN IMAGERY USING A DIRECTIONALLY SELECTIVE LOCAL FEATURE STATISTICS OPERATOR

DUNCAN TELFER [†],

Department of Computing, University of Central Lancashire, Preston, PR1 2HE, UK

[†] Current Address: *Centre for Intelligent Monitoring Systems*, Department of Electrical Engineering and Electronics, University of Liverpool, L69 3GJ, UK*
e-mail : djtelfer@liverpool.ac.uk
* CIMS@liv.ac.uk

A texture discrimination scheme based on combining directional outputs from a local feature statistics operator is described. The method is an extension of that of Telfer and Pritchard[2] with improved isotropy and directional resolution, and has been applied to woodgrain test images from the album of Brodatz[1] to assess its applicability for mapping woodgrain textures and their directional deviance. Textures of interest are compared with a user-selected reference window. Histograms are generated of local texture features within windowed regions for auto-correlation with the output from the reference window. Through directionally resolved segmentation, it is possible to quantify changes in texture alignment within the image field. The results for images of several types of woodgrain textures demonstrate the potential of the method for automated inspection of timber surfaces. This suggests that the approach can be the basis for a promising quality control tool.
Keywords. *Image processing, mask operator, texture segmentation, automated inspection, woodgrain.*

1   Introduction.

Textures in general may be classified for convenience as deterministic, e.g., the predictable geometric pattern of a chess board; stochastic, i.e., predominantly noise, and thirdly, structural, in which there are observable small scale geometric features which may repeat but are not necessarily identical over the textured region; e.g., a pebbled beach, tree bark, grass and foliage. The observable features often include directional bias, as in most woodgrains. In cases where constancy of directional alignment of the grain is important, e.g., in structural timber, a means of quantifying deviation from alignment could assist in timber selection and product quality control.

The goal of the image processing procedure reported in this paper is to demarcate, or map, the spatial distribution of a particular texture type in digitised images of woodgrains. Image regions with identifiable textural differences are generally readily perceived and this is the usual starting point for motivating the processing of a particular image. In this work, the images were processed off-line, and image selection was guided by necessity to provide a context for the application of the technique. Monochrome (grey-range 0..255) images were used, at a spatial resolution of 512 x 512 pixels.

Telfer and Pritchard[2] reported a windowed correlation scheme using a 2x2 local difference operator, which responded well to fields containing structured textures, whereas the 'classical' windowed grey-level histogram correlation technique was more useful for discriminating between stochastic texture fields. Their paper acknowledged that while directionality was a significant textural property, in remote sensing terrain images it is often required to ignore distinctions attributable to direction dependence.

The scheme in this work had significant enhancements, in that it encoded 16 rather than 8 directions, also with improved isotropy of response.

Here, window size was changed from 25x25 (square) to 30 pixels diameter (circular). The increased image resolution, from 256x256 pixels to 512x512, permitted use of a larger local difference operator needed for the increased angular resolution. The operator mask size was increased from 2x2 pixels to 7x7, arguably with some risk in undersampling the image contents. But with suitable choices of window placement and digitisation scale for the subject, this problem can be mitigated.

2 Autocorrelation method.

In this work, the example mask structures in Fig. 1 show how the mask elements E are labelled in a power of two series 1..128. Local differences between image pixels under opposite elements were used to accumulate a unique 8-bit code value for each of 16 mask directions. For example, if the pixel under E2 is greater than that under

E64 then the accumulator is incremented by 64, and so on, for each of the 4 element pairs. This was repeated for rotations of the masks to give 16 possible directions, allowing response to correspondingly rotated textures. Clearly, square tessellation brings about slight non-equivalence in geometry (Fig.1) between the two sets of masks. For each mask direction, a histogram of these local neighborhood encodings was constructed over a reference window taken from a texture of interest in the image. Each of the selected directional histograms for the reference window was then compared with histograms in a single (principal) direction for windows scanned at one pixel intervals over the whole image. For a given image, the resulting auto-correlation coefficients were normalised to a scale 0.255 for display as correlation maps. For our purposes, only 6 directions were 'turned on' in the output, as shown in Fig. 2b.

3 The mask operators.

At the mask level, the objective is to create a code value which is the index into a histogram array, the indexed element to be incremented by 1. The 8-bit code is generated from eight local pixel differences according to an arbitrary but fixed scheme as shown in Fig. 1, which gives four examples from the series of 16 masks. These masks are of two types. The symmetrical type (Figs. 1b, d) accommodates relative texture orientations at 0, 90, 180 and 270 degrees, and the diagonals between; the asymmetric type (Figs. 1a, c) are assigned to each of the directions which bisect the 45 degree sectors bounded by the orientation axes for the symmetrical masks. The direction giving the maximum output is selected for plotting a normalised correlation map (integer, range 0..255).

4 Practical considerations.

Four main problems can be identified: {1} the illumination of the target may be such that the rotation of a texture field in the plane of the image affects the reflectance pattern; {2} the effects of spatial quantisation in square tessellation may give rise to differences in rendering of a given texture for different directions; a further difficulty {3} is also associated with spatial quantisation and involves the geometric non-equivalence of the mask elements along different axes of four-fold symmetry. Lastly {4}, depending on the complexity of image contents, ambiguities may arise in the output; the aggregate of local operator outputs contributing to a histogram from within a window may generate a similar histogram for different perceived textures. Problem {1} is extrinsic and largely beyond the control of the image processing procedure. Problem {2} may be tackled at the pre-digitisation stage by scanning or photographing the scene itself in different directions. In this work, no attempt at such correction was found necessary. Problem {3} would have been a significant impediment to achieving isotropy with a 2x2 mask, but was much less problematic with the 7x7 configurations used here. Problem {4} could be tackled by using more combinations of local differences (increased coding range). For example, Wang and He[3] assigned over 6000 combinations or 'texture unit' primitives using a 3x3 pixel mask, but in order to generate reasonably well populated histograms for the windows, a histogram size of 256 bins is retained for this work.

5 Output using the 'rings' test image.

Fig. 2a shows a test pattern with graduated sets of concentric rings at five different scales. The gray-level radial cross-sections are sawtooth in profile. This confers unambiguous directionality on opposite sides of the image. The image is 512x512 pixels spatial resolution at 256 grey levels. The reference window is positioned at x=400, y=400 (origin at top left) and yields the 16-direction response in Fig. 2b. The thresholded output is grey-level coded to show the angular responses of interest in this work. The grey-tone coding scheme is as follows for the six tones g0..g5 (dark..light) with g6 as white (Table 1).

TABLE 1. Threshold encodings for directions. [These may be arbitrary to suit the viewer].

Grey-Tone (Figs. 2, 3b, 4b, 5b)   Relative axis alignment   Colour (Fig.7)

Grey-Tone		Relative axis alignment	Colour
g0	darkest grey	principal axis forward	dark blue
g1		principal axis reverse	mid blue
g2		+ 22.5 deg. forward	cyan
g3		+ 22.5 deg. reverse	green
g4		- 22.5 deg. forward	yellow
g5	lightest grey	- 22.5 deg. reverse	orange
g6	white (background)	other directions	red

The other response lobes in Fig 2b. were switched off in the displayed output of these texture deviation experiments.

Many natural textures have bilateral symmetry, so that the forward and reverse responses can often be grouped together. But they are separated here to reveal underlying structure in the output images.

6 Results: woodgrain textures.

The new local differences operator showed clearly the departure from the texture alignment in the reference window taken for each of the following Brodatz textures.

Maple, #WW3, Fig. 3a. The reference window encloses two dark bars at low resolution, along with relatively indistinct elongated micro-features in mainly horizontal orientation. In Fig. 3b, a sharp cut-off beyond the region responding to the –22.5 degree forward/reverse lobes is evident, as is the demarcation boundary with response from the lobes on the principal axis. Also, the banded structure in the forward/reverse responses frequently continues across this boundary.

Oak, #WW19, Fig 4a. Here, the reference window encloses horizontal-running fine grain features but undersamples the growth-ring pattern. In Fig. 4b, the output is dominated by response to these fine-grain features, as is evidenced by the sparse response in the upper parts of the texture map. The growth-ring pattern exerts some influence, however, as is shown by the +22.5 response just above centre left.

Mahogany, #WW23. Fig. 4b. In this example, the fine-grain texture is totally dominant. Here we return to an unambiguous demarcation boundary with the +22.5 degree (relative) region in the lower third of the image. There are some very low frequency modulations, some of which attenuate the texture and elsewhere affect its alignment (note the localised −25.5 degree response above centre right); although interesting, these are relatively minor effects. Of more significance is the thin ribbon-like 'no-man's land' response between the two main directional regions. This might be attributable to the texture in this zone falling between the two angular responses; but it does not occur in Fig. 3b and suggests the need for further ongoing work with test imagery.

The discrimination capability was compared to a scheme using a 3x3 Kirsch operator, the directional output being labelled 0..7 and the parametric image obtained further processed by again taking 30x30 windows and creating histograms (with bins 0..7) from the directional data. The windowed raw histogram data was then compared with that from the reference window (using the same sets of reference window coordinates) to produce correlation maps for the Kirsch directions (Fig. 6). There is significantly less discrimination capability and revealed structural content in the Kirsch maps.

Fig. 7a is a 3D brightness profile rendering of the output image in Fig. 3b using the 3DEM display package (R.S. Horne ©1995, 1997). Fig. 7b is the corresponding rendering of Fig. 5b.

7 Summary and conclusions.

Isotropic and directionally separable texture discrimination using 7x7 masks operators in 16 orientations for generating histograms of encoded directional differencing of image pixels under the mask elements has been applied to test images and woodgrain imagery from the Brodatz 1971 album. Successful discrimination at axial resolution of +/- 22.5 degrees suggests that implementation of the isotropic operator would be a useful basis for selection/rejection of timber on the basis of angular deviation of the woodgrain pattern.

8 Acknowledgements.

Software was developed in Pascal and Ada for running on Pentium PCs. Thanks are due the University of of Central Lancashire for provision of computing facilities for the Texture99 version of this paper, and to the University of Liverpool during this revision.

9 References.

1. Brodatz, P.,1971. Texture: Woodgrains. A Photographic Album for Artists and Designers. Dover, NY.
2. Telfer, D.J. and Pritchard, K.O., 1995. Histogram correlation of the output from a small mask operator: A basis for adaptive texture segmentation. *Proc. 5th IEE Int. Conf. on Image Processing and its Applications.Edinburgh.*
3. Wang, L. and He, D-C., 1989. A new statistical approach for texture analysis. *Amer. Soc. Photogrammetry and Remote Sensing, Image Processing, '89, Sparks, Nevada.*

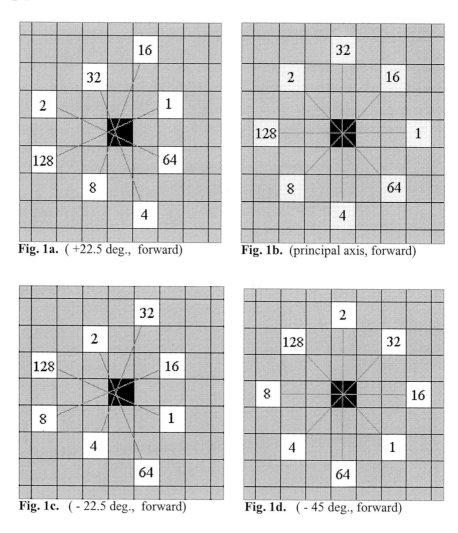

Fig. 1a. (+22.5 deg., forward)   **Fig. 1b.** (principal axis, forward)

Fig. 1c. (- 22.5 deg., forward)   **Fig. 1d.** (- 45 deg., forward)

Legend:

Part of the series of 16 masks for the 7x7 local difference operator. The position labels rotate progressively through the series in nominally 22.5 degree steps, given the slight geometric distortions inherent in the odd-numbered masks due to the limitations imposed by quantisation.

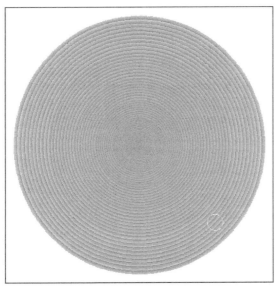

Fig2a. 'Rings' test image containing graduated concentric ramps.
The reference region (30 pixels dia.) is circled.

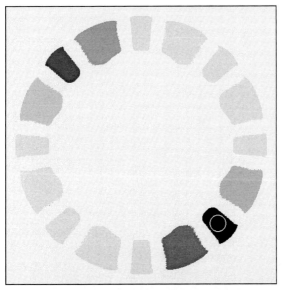

Fig. 2b. Response pattern of 16-direction algorithm to the 'Rings'
image. The six principal lobes of interest (darkest texture orientation
directions) are grey-level coded as shown above. Responses from
the other lobes are ignored in the texture deviation experiments.

248

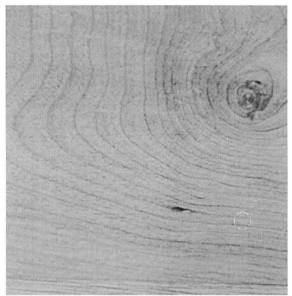

Fig. 3a. Maple, Cat # WW3 (Brodatz, 1971). Reference window circled.

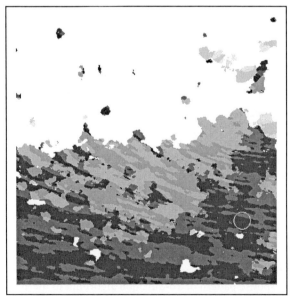

Fig. 3b. WW3 texture map showing directional deviation (see text).

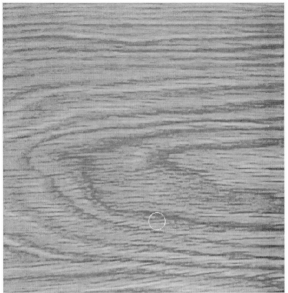

Fig. 4a. Oak, Cat # WW19

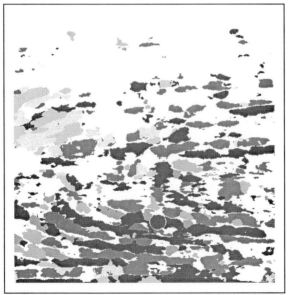

Fig. 4b. WW19 texture map. The output is dominated by response to fine-grain features within the window of Fig. 4a (see text).

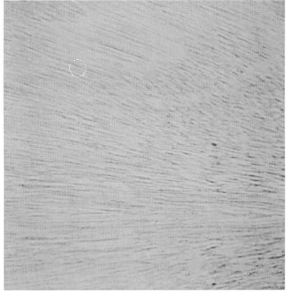

Fig. 5a. Mahogany burl. Cat # WW23.

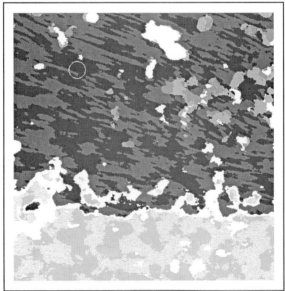

Fig. 5b. WW23 texture map illustrating 'contoured' response to gradual change in texture direction.

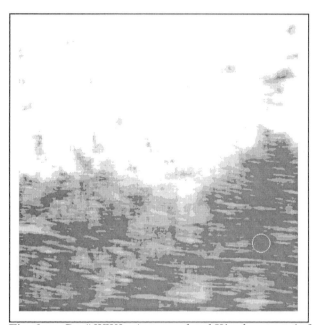

Fig. 6a. Cat # WW3. Autocorrelated Kirsch output (c.f., Fig. 3b.)

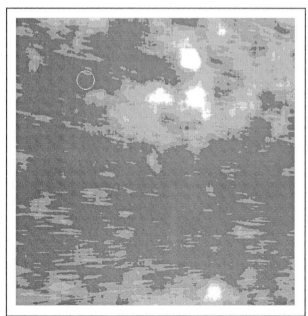

Fig. 6b. Cat #WW23. Autocorrelated Kirsch output (c.f., Fig. 5b).

252

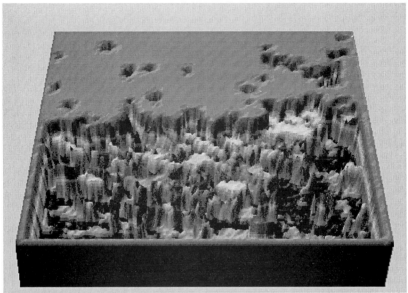

Fig. 7a. Maple, Cat # WW3. 3DEM™ rendered version of Fig. 3b.

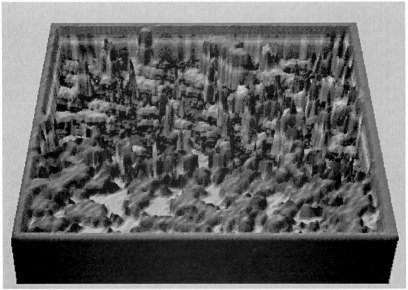

Fig. 7b. Mahogany Cat # WW23. 3DEM™ rendering of Fig. 5b.

COMBINING ANALYSIS AND SYNTHESIS OF TEXTURES FOR THE ANIMATION INDUSTRY

MARK OLLILA, ANDERS JACKSON, AND AARON ARDIRI

Creative Media Lab, University of Gävle, SE-801 76, Gävle, Sweden

E-mail: {molly,jackson,ardiri}@hig.se

We examine the use of genetic algorithms for the synthesis of textures based on aesthetic judgements of a human user. A set of genes, describing various mathematical operators and functions, are used to generate an expression tree which is used to determine the final texture. These genes are cross-bred, mutated, and new populations generated according to the selections of a human user. This paper examines the design and implementation of a system based on the analysis and synthesis of textures, in particularly, for practical use in the animation industry.

1   Introduction

In the animation industry, texture synthesis and analysis is an important part of everyday work. Normally, real textures are gathered and scanned, and then modified by artists. Alternatively, artists spend hours generating the necessary textures by hand. Both processes often involve tedious work before the final texture is ready to be used in production. It should be remembered that the final texture generated might often be used in both photorealistic and non-photorealistic productions, and hence deal with both natural, artificial, and unreal textures.

Traditional approaches to the texture synthesis problem have often used color information and texture features for image interpretation. Textures are often expressed as a set of regular patterns, themselves consisting of a set of elementary components (texels). In macro-textures, the texture primitives themselves have significant features as well as some form of spatial arrangement. Micro-textures, on the other hand, are patterns with small primitives, which in the extreme case consist of only single pixels. Statistical models are particularly suited for modelling micro-textures [3,6,13].

When dealing with color, there have been two traditional approaches, that of single-channel texture analysis and multi-channel texture analysis. In single-color texture analysis, extraction of texture features is performed separately in each color channel. With multi-channel texture analysis the interrelations between different color channels are considered [14]. The spatial arrangements of colors are described in different approaches which are based on second order statistics, such as co-occurrence matrices or Markov random field texture model [12]. Histogram techniques have also been used for the synthesis of textures by iteratively alternating between matching the sub-band histograms and matching pixel histograms of the images [7].

What we examine here is how the previous texture analysis and synthesis techniques could be used in the animation industry. In particular, we want to design a solution which combines the animators ability to judge an aesthetically pleasing texture, with the ability to design new ones. Artists and animators are usually not interested in the mathematical parameterizations of a texture or the method used in the synthesis. They realize that there are problems with current synthesis techniques, as there are problems with scanned images of real textures. These might include the finite size and resolution, the lighting, and also the tiling of the texture across a surface may also cause unnatural periodicity. To defeat this, it has been suggested that writing shaders (programmes that generate textures) might seem to be a powerful approach, but in practice it is often very difficult to achieve the desired look. Artists are often the people involved with deciding the look and feel of a texture for a particular scene in the animation industry, and often are not well versed in the mathematical nature of textures. It is due to this problem, that this system, based on a concept of genetic textures (GENTEX) is been developed.

2   System Design

The system generates procedural textures using techniques from the artificial intelligence literature. The system operates in both a human-in-the-loop (for example, the animator/artist) and automatic texture matching modes. In human-in-the-loop mode, the user controls the aesthetic and parametric evaluation and selection. These parameters might include symmetry, color, local structure, global structure, and similarities. The particular question of aesthetics is a parameter that will vary amongst animators themselves, and often requires further definition. This process of shaping a texture interactively (through an iterative process) will often involve some chance. The issue of chance in image assessments was presented by Squire and Pun [16] with respect to the machine and human assessments of the organization of images in image databases. This is important when designing an automatic (machine driven) mode for texture synthesis based on aesthetics in that the appearance of intelligent selection, could actually be purely random.

In automatic mode, the system compares rendered images of generated textures to images of target textures, using texture matching techniques often used in the computer vision literature [6,11].

The system extends research performed previously using artificial intelligence techniques as shown by Sims [15] and by Ibrahim and House [8]. In using genetic algorithms, a population of textures is obtained by examining a predefined library of textures, testing these images from the textures against the target texture and scoring the images. This is similar to the image database problem. Alternatively, the system can begin by randomly generating a population from a pool of genes. The scoring of the images is done via a fitness function which ranks the current parameters and how successful the match is with respect to the qualities that the animator/artist has chosen. The system selects the initial population from that receiving the best scores. Selection in the interactive mode is similar but based on the user's aesthetic judgement.

Parent textures are selected and bred to create new children for the ongoing population. When breeding two hierarchies of textures, the breeding procedure selects a random node in each hierarchy and swaps the subtrees under these nodes. This is known as crossover in the genetic algorithm literature. The system evaluates images of generated textures in automatic mode, while in interactive mode the human user scores the images of textures based on their aesthetic judgement. The new population of images are generated using a genetic algorithm which is used to determine which textures will survive.

After a new population is generated, using, the interactive mode, users repeat the previous steps to generate a new population and so on until they are satisfied with the result, both aesthetically and technically. In the automatic mode, the generation continues until a generated texture is sufficiently close to the target texture or a maximum number of generations have been reached. Random mutation is used to introduce diversity into the population.

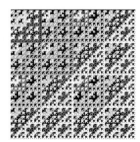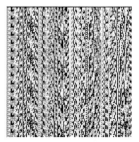

Figure 1: Some sample textures synthesized from a gene pool of 19 genes.

Neural network techniques are examined to help guide the genetic algorithms in deciding if the current population is suitable for evolution, mutation, or if a crossover is required for instance, as well as in the analysis of the results [17].

3   Current Research Problems

A few recent systems do exist that attempt to solve the synthesis problem, either using covariance based techniques [9], or using some simplified form of decision theory or artificial intelligence [8]. Problems that exist in current research in the area include over simplified fitness functions, not enough suitable gene representations, and lack of aesthetics in the guidance of evolution. There is also a need to merge the three problems of image retrieval, image analysis, and image synthesis together. This is particularly the case when we look at the animation industry where texture databases do exist. The synthesis problem could therefore be reduced down to an image similarity retrieval problem. This, in conjunction with the ability to analyse a texture, followed by generating variations of it, is a useful tool for the animation industry.

The problems that need to be solved in the near future include how features (both local and global) are represented as genes and then evolved. The current implementation of GENTEX uses a tree structure, but more complicated, two dimensional representations need to be examined [2]. The ability to compress and optimize the current expression tree that represents the texture is also required.

To solve these problems, artificial intelligence techniques used together with standard techniques are required. This means incorporating technologies such as neural networks; evolutionary programming, intelligent agents in combination with traditional covariance/statistical based methods. Another approach is to perform automated reasoning with feedback to guide the design of the shaders [10,11].

4   Conclusions

The use of artificial intelligence techniques in the generation of textures, in both analysis and synthesis, is of great practical importance for the animation industry. The techniques examined include genetic algorithms and how these are combined with traditional methods of texture synthesis. The results from this research will help in the development of tools and technologies that can generate the feeling in the audience that there is no distinction between the film and the animation. If this achieved, then there is more freedom for the animator and the film director in future productions. This is an important consequence from this research.

5   Acknowledgements

The authors were partially supported by a grant by KK-Stiftelsens Dnr. 1997/1294 and funding from Commando Royale AB. Students Erik Lindqvist and Rickard Lindqvist worked on this project as part of their course work.

References.

1. Caelli T. and Ollila M., In-place covariance operators for computer vision. In *ICIAP95*, San Remo, September 1995.
2. Cartwright H.M. and Harris S.P., The application of the genetic algorithm to two-dimensional strings: the source apportionment problem, in *Int. Conf.. on Genetic Algorithms*, Urbana-Champaign, IL, 1993.
3. Cross G. and Jain A., Markov random field texture models. *IEEE Transactions on Pattern Analysis and Machine Intelligence (PAMI)*, Vol 5., pp 25-39, 1983.
4. Ebert D.S., Texture and Modeling. A Procedural Approach. 1994. Academic Press.
5. Healey G. and Wang L., Illumination-invariant recognition of texture in color images, *Journal of the Optical Society of America*, Vol. 12, No. 9. 1995. pp 1877-1883.
6. Haralick R.M., Statistical and Structural Approaches to Texture, *Proc. Of the IEEE*, Vol. 67, 1979. pp. 786-804
7. Heeger D. and Bergen J., Pyramid-based texture analysis/synthesis. In *Proc. ACM SIGGRAPH*, August 1995.
8. Ibrahim A.M. and House D.H., Genetic Shaders: Interactive and Automatic Shader Generation. 1997. *SIGGRAPH* 1997 Sketch.
9. Lakmann R. and Priese L., A Reduced Covariance Color Texture Model for Micro-Textures. In 10th *Scandinavian Conference on Image Analysis*, Finland, 1997. pp 947-953.
10. Ollila M. and Caelli T., Automatic geometric reasoning using algebraic methods with image processing techniques. In *WACSS94*, Perth, September 1994.
11. Ollila M. and Caelli T., Networking of geometric concepts for algebraic metrology. In *ACCV 95*, Singapore, December 1995.
12. Panjwani D.K and Healey G., Markov random field models for unsupervised segmentation of textured color images, *IEEE Transactions on Pattern Analysis and Machine Intelligence (PAMI)*, Vol. 17. No 10. 1995, pp. 939-954.
13. Reed T.R. and Du Buf J.M.H., A review of recent texture segmentation and feature extraction techniques, *CVGIP: Image Understanding*, Vol. 57. No. 3. 1993. pp. 359-372.
14. Scharcanski J., Hovis J.K., and Shen H.C., Representing the color aspect of texture images, *Pattern Recognition Letters*, Vol. 15, 1994, pp. 191-197.
15. Sims K., Artificial Evolution for Computer Graphics. *Computer graphics*, Vol. 25, 4. July 1991.
16. Squire D. McG. and Pun T., A Comparison of Human and Machine Assessments of Image Similarity for the Organization of Image Databases. *Scandinavian Conference on Image Analysis*. June 9-11, 1997, Lappeenranta, Finland.

17. Wiles J. and Ollila M., Intersecting regions: the key to combinatorial structure in hidden unit space. In *Neural Information Processing Systems 5*, 5, Denver, December 1992.

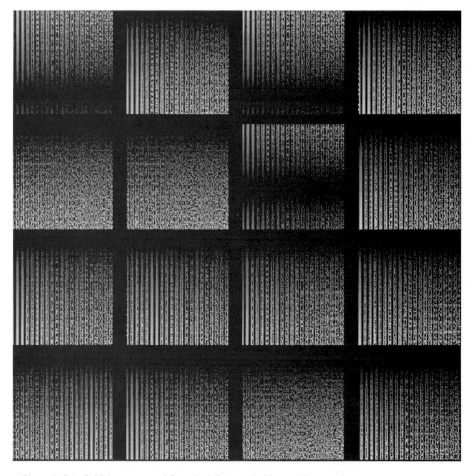

Figure 2: Set of children generated from the left parent in Figure 1. by mutation.

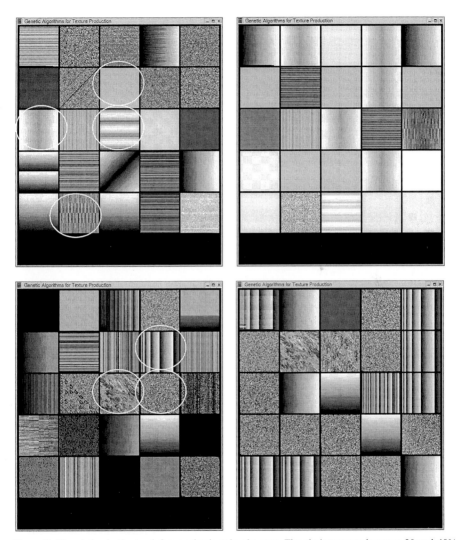

Figure 3: The circles in the top left are selections by the user. The choices range between 20 and 40% satisfaction. The next generation based on this is presented. The next example shows one texture with 70% satisfactions with two others at 20%. The resulting generation is then presented to the right.

COLOR FIGURES

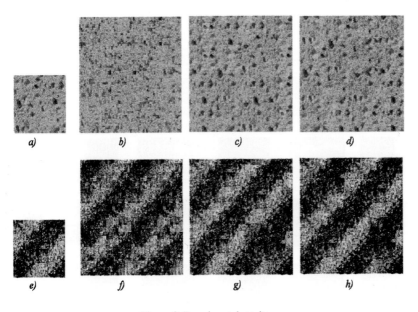

a)   b)   c)   d)

e)   f)   g)   h)

Figure 3. Experimental results.

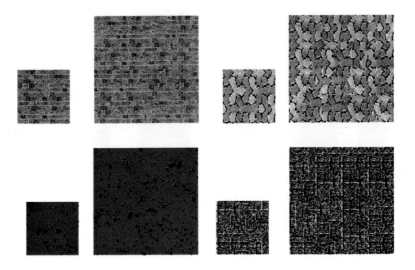

Figure 4. Further experimental results obtained with the mixed approach.

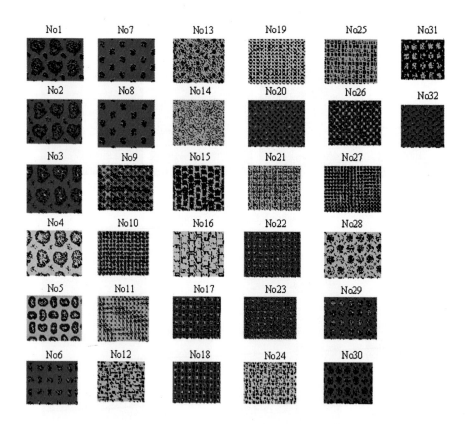

Figure 1. 32 colour patterns

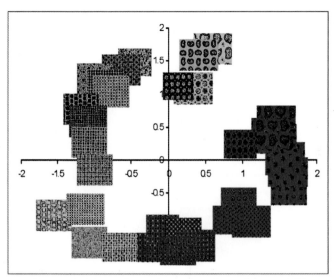

Figure 3. 2D-configuration points from observer DH

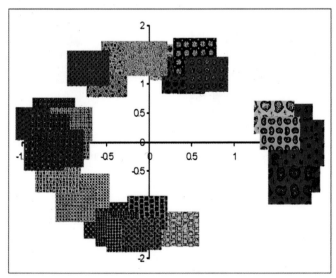

Figure 4. 2D-configuration points from observer CR

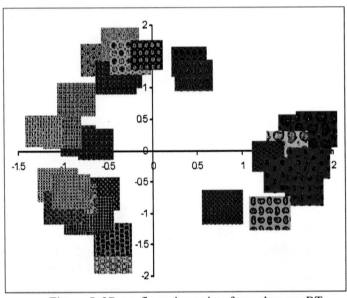

Figure 5. 2D-configuration points from observer BT

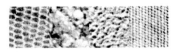

Figure 7. Brodatz texture images.

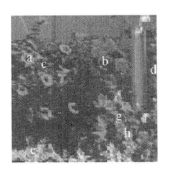

Figure 5. Test image.

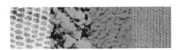

Figure 8. Texture coloring.

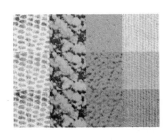

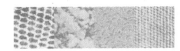

Figure 9. Texture coloring (fixed μ).

Figure 6. Coloring (small color difference).

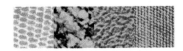

Figure 10. Texture coloring (fixed σ).

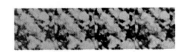

Figure 11. Coloring, $\alpha = 1(\text{left}), 0.8, 0.5, 0$.

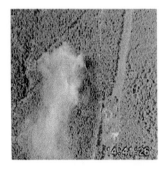

Figure 12. Color image.

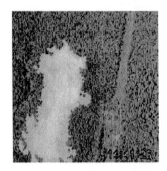

Figure 13. Coloring, spruce spectrum, $\gamma = 0.4$.

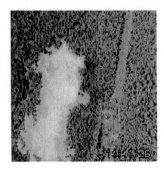

Figure 14. Coloring, birch spectrum, $\gamma = 0.55$.

VI

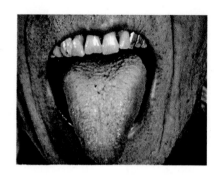

Figure 3: Tongue Image (colour)

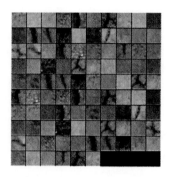

Figure 4: Reference Textures

TTB

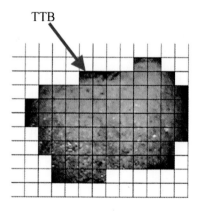

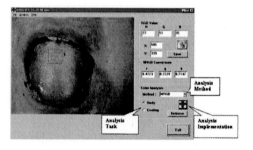

Figure 5: Selected TTBs to be analyzed   Figure 6: A tongue diagnosis interface

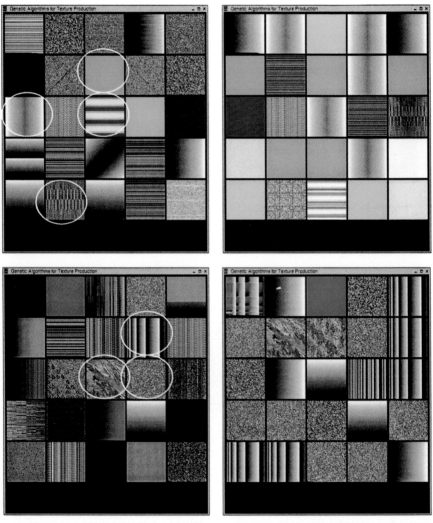

Figure 3: The circles in the top left are selections by the user. The choices range between 20 and 40% satisfaction. The next generation based on this is presented. The next example shows one texture with 70% satisfactions with two others at 20%. The resulting generation is then presented to the right.